THE WAR
AGAINST
VIRUSES

Also by Aileen Burford-Mason

The Healthy Brain

Eat Well, Age Better

THE WAR AGAINST VIRUSES

HOW THE SCIENCE OF OPTIMAL NUTRITION CAN HELP YOU WIN

AILEEN BURFORD-MASON

PATRICK CREAN EDITIONS
HarperCollins*Publishers*Ltd

For my friends Sampa Bhadra and John Martin

Published by Patrick Crean Editions, an imprint of HarperCollins Publishers Ltd

First edition

This book contains advice and information relating to health care. It should be used to supplement rather
than replace the advice of your doctor or another trained health professional. If you know or suspect that
you have a health problem, it is recommended that you seek your physician's advice before embarking on
any diet or supplement regime. All efforts have been made to assure the accuracy of the information
contained in this book as of the date of publication. The publisher and the author disclaim liability for
any medical outcomes that may occur as a result of applying the methods suggested in this book.

HarperCollins books may be purchased for educational, business,
or sales promotional use through our Special Markets Department.

HarperCollins Publishers Ltd
Bay Adelaide Centre, East Tower
22 Adelaide Street West, 41st Floor
Toronto, Ontario, Canada
M5H 4E3

www.harpercollins.ca

Library and Archives Canada Cataloguing in Publication

Title: The war against viruses : how the science of optimal nutrition can help you win /
Aileen Burford-Mason.
Names: Burford-Mason, Aileen, author.
Description: First edition. | Includes bibliographical references.
Identifiers: Canadiana (print) 20210143401 | Canadiana (ebook) 20210143800 | ISBN
9781443463270 (softcover) | ISBN 9781443463287 (ebook)
Subjects: LCSH: Immunity—Nutritional aspects—Popular works. | LCSH: Immune system—
Popular works. | LCSH: Orthomolecular therapy—Popular works. | LCSH: Dietary supplements—
Popular works. | LCSH: Virus diseases—Popular works.
Classification: LCC QR182.2.N86 B87 2021 | DDC 616.07/9—dc23

Printed and bound in the United States of America
21 22 23 24 LSC 10 9 8 7 6 5 4 3 2 1

CONTENTS

INTRODUCTION

In June 2019, I was in Vancouver to speak at a conference. My talk was on immunity and susceptibility to colds and flu, and it married two major interests of mine: the immune system and its workings, and nutrition. During the talk, I focused on the reliance of the immune system on a healthy diet. If the immune system malfunctioned, I suggested, maybe inadequate diets had something to do with it.

Towards the end of my talk, I raised the possibility that, sooner or later, we would be faced with an extremely contagious infection that could rampage across the world and cause many to fall seriously ill. Not an original idea. For some years, scientists had been sounding the alarm that a major pandemic, similar in magnitude to the Spanish flu of 1918–19, was likely, if not inevitable. In March 2020, the World Health Organization (WHO) classified a new fast-moving viral infection named COVID-19 as a pandemic.

As the pandemic unfolded, it became obvious that people were drowning in information, bombarded with new concepts and terminologies that were unfamiliar; that the lack of a basic knowledge framework with which to understand this crisis was adding to everyone's anxieties. So many questions needed answering: What were the key components of the immune system, and how exactly did it work? What was so special about this new virus that it was a threat to global health?

For my part, I was concerned that there was so little discussion around nutrition and the vital role it played in supporting our immune systems, despite the fact that poor diets and chronically low intakes of nutrients like vitamin D had long been known to compromise our ability to fight infection. Missing from the public health debate was any notion that nutritional strategies might be helpful in the fight against COVID-19.

And so the concept for this book took shape. Although written against a backdrop of COVID-19, the book is not intended as a blow-by-blow account of the pandemic's first year. At the time of writing, the pandemic shows no sign of abating, and a complete telling of its story may not be written for many years. Neither does this book aim to be a comprehensive primer on viruses or the immune system—that would be an impossible task to accomplish coherently in one book. I simply want to give the reader enough information to understand why viruses pose a particular threat to health, and how, in battling them, our immune systems either work to our advantage or turn against us, causing us harm.

The nutritional strategies outlined in this book not only provide a recipe for improved health in general, but could go a long way towards improving immune health. Since scientists predict that this may not be the last pandemic we will be exposed to in our lifetimes, correcting nutritional inadequacies should provide enhanced immune support in advance of being exposed to any new and potentially lethal infections.

Aileen Burford-Mason

January 2021

PART I

AN INVISIBLE ENEMY

CHAPTER ONE

An Ill-Prepared World

The world is ill prepared to respond to an influenza pandemic or any similar global, sustained and threatening public health emergency.
—*World Health Organization: Sixty-Fourth World Health Assembly, May 5, 2011*[1]

It's New Year's Eve 2019 and the party is in full swing. I've spent the evening with a group of lively friends in Toronto, sharing food and drink and generally making merry. All evening, the wine has flowed freely and everyone is in high spirits. Some are dancing, others are sharing their New Year's resolutions, which mostly appear to revolve around plans to improve health and fitness in the coming year—to lose those extra ten pounds that somehow crept up over the previous twelve months; to exercise more and give up alcohol—at least for the month of January.

Around the world, this ancient celebration—ringing out the old year and bringing in the new—is steeped in significance. It's a time of reflection; a time for resetting goals and aspirations. It's a time to be upbeat and optimistic—we've made it through the last 365 days relatively unscathed and are eager to see what's in store for us in the coming year.

Our hosts distribute flutes of champagne. Someone puts the TV on and we watch the festivities unfold in front of City Hall as the countdown begins. Exactly at midnight, the sky over Toronto fills with fireworks. Everyone exchanges hugs and kisses. Happy New Year, we wish each other. Hope it's a great one!

But 2020 would not be the year we anticipated—not by a long shot. Rather than the health and happiness we were hoping for, we were about to enter a collective health crisis the likes of which the world had not experienced in a hundred years.

DECEMBER 31 IN CHINA

On the same day, on the other side of the world, the Chinese government was officially preparing to alert the World Health Organization to a worrisome outbreak of viral pneumonia occurring in Wuhan—a city of eleven million inhabitants and the largest transport hub in central China. The infection appeared to have started in a busy "wet market"—a food market where live animals were bought and then killed on site for food. Wet markets were known breeding grounds for infection, and the Chinese government had repeatedly but unsuccessfully tried to shut them down. The close proximity of the animals—often wild or exotic—kept stacked in cages, together with poor hygiene at the market, allowed for easy transmission of disease from animal to animal. From time to time those infections jumped from animals to humans.

The outbreak quickly escalated, and within a few weeks 262 cities in China had reported cases. On January 23, two days before the Chinese New Year, the government declared the outbreak a national emergency. Concerned that the massive exodus of citizens from Wuhan during the New Year would further spread the infection, all transport in and out of the city was stopped. Suspected and confirmed cases were isolated, bus and subway travel suspended, schools and entertainment venues closed and public gatherings banned.

It would later transpire that the Chinese government had been reluctant to alert the world to the real scale and contagious nature of this new infection, and that they had silenced scientists who earlier had tried to raise the alarm. The most important fact—that the virus was not only acquired by contact with infected animals, but was easily spread from person to person—would only gradually emerge. Governments everywhere were therefore slow in implementing travel bans to and from China, until it was too late. The horse was out of the starting gate and widespread dissemination of the virus, first to Europe and then progressively around the world, had already happened.

On January 13, the WHO declared the outbreak a "public health emergency of international concern." As winter drifted into spring, the full magnitude of the outbreak became obvious. By early March, the outbreak was so widespread that the WHO declared that it now met all the criteria for a pandemic. Over the next weeks, country after country went into lockdown. Efforts to stop community spread included travel bans within and between countries, and mandatory quarantine of symptomatic individuals and anyone they had been in contact with.

Workplaces were shuttered, schools and places of worship were closed and people were instructed to stay at home, unless they needed to shop for food or medicine. No inviting your neighbour in for a cup of coffee and a chat; no hugging and kissing or handshakes. Social distancing—maintaining a two-metre or six-foot space between individuals—became the new norm.

Despite early measures aimed at containment, the death rate rose relentlessly. In the worst-hit areas, makeshift hospitals sprouted in parking lots, open fields and city parks. Refrigerated trucks were pressed into use as temporary morgues to house the dead. As an article in the *British Medical Journal* expressed it, the world as we knew it was "being destroyed by a pathogen spreading with the ruthless vengeance of a Biblical plague."[2]

GETTING TO KNOW THE ENEMY

The pathogen causing all this trouble was quickly identified as a member of a large group of viruses called coronaviruses—so named because, under the electron microscope, spikes on the outer coat of the viruses looked rather like a crown. The WHO named the new coronavirus SARS-COV2, and the disease it caused COVID-19, to reflect the year the virus first appeared.

Science had been aware of coronaviruses since the 1930s, mainly as a cause of serious gastrointestinal or respiratory infections in animals. From time to time, a coronavirus would emerge that wreaked havoc in agricultural livestock. One of them caused severe diarrhea and widespread death in baby pigs. Another was known to cause a bronchitis-like illness in chickens. Coronaviruses had even occasionally been shown to be the cause of death when dead beluga whales washed up on shore.

But although this particular class of viruses was of concern in the veterinary world, they appeared to be relatively harmless in humans. Certainly, four coronaviruses had been identified in the 1960s that were responsible for 10 to 15 per cent of seasonal colds (the rest being caused by one or another of a swarm of viruses that orbit around us each winter).[3] But these illnesses were generally mild and self-limiting, so developing treatments to prevent or treat them wasn't a medical priority.

Then, in 2002, the medical community was taken off guard by the emergence of a new coronavirus that was much more serious than the common cold. Known by the acronym SARS (severe acute respiratory syndrome) and starting in southern China, its origin was also thought to have been a wet market, and that it perhaps had transmitted from bats to civet cats, and then to humans. SARS spread rapidly outside China and eventually affected twenty-six countries. Over eight thousand people were infected. About 10 per cent of those who contracted the virus died.

In 2012, a second serious coronavirus showed up: Middle East respiratory syndrome, or MERS. Originally observed in Saudi Arabia, MERS too had started in animals and was believed to have been transmitted to humans from camels. Like SARS, MERS became pandemic, eventually spreading to twenty-six other countries. The WHO reported roughly 2,500 cases worldwide. At 34 per cent, the fatality rate from MERS was significantly higher than that of SARS.[4]

Although SARS and MERS were different coronaviruses, the symptoms they caused were very similar. They would begin with a fever and other flu-like symptoms and quickly progress to a dry cough and extreme shortness of breath. Typically more severe in patients already being treated for other conditions such as heart disease or diabetes,[5] there was no treatment, and since these were novel viruses, no protective vaccine.

COVID-19: FROM MILD INCONVENIENCE TO FATAL DISEASE

Unlike with SARS and MERS, most of those who got COVID-19 experienced only minor symptoms, similar to a cold or flu. Some had no symptoms at all. WHO's director general, Tedros Adhanom Ghebreyesus, predicted that more than 80 per cent of patients who acquired COVID-19 would have a "mild disease and will recover." But for the 20 per cent who got more serious disease, COVID-19 was like nothing else they had ever experienced. Not like a cold; not like the flu.

Just like SARS and MERS, the infection would begin with flu-like symptoms: fever, a cough and sometimes body aches, and in some but not all patients, progress to extreme shortness of breath and a profound fatigue. The cough was a hard, dry paroxysmal cough, attacks of which could be so bad, they frequently caused vomiting. "You feel like you're going to die," recovered patients frequently reported. Some patients needed to be hospitalized; others were told just to self-quarantine and battle it out at home—isolating themselves from other family members, resting, drinking lots of fluids and hoping they would recover without a trip to their nearest hospital emergency department.

In the US, New York City became a hot spot for COVID-19. By early April, the virus had killed three times more citizens than the terrifying terrorist attacks on the World Trade Center on September 11, 2001 (9/11), previously considered the greatest disaster the city had experienced in modern memory. Day by day, the number of infections and fatalities escalated at an alarming rate. New Yorkers listened in disbelief as New York governor Andrew Cuomo pleaded for undertakers to be drafted in from other states to help them bury their dead.

Seniors appeared to be the most vulnerable, and children seemed mercifully spared—or at least experienced only mild symptoms. Nursing homes, long-term care facilities and retirement residences were particularly hard hit. This was no surprise, really. The elderly—often frail and already at high risk of dying from pneumonia and the milder seasonal flu—were cocooned in close quarters, ideal targets for infection. When the body count was finally in, nursing home deaths would account for up to 80 per cent of total deaths worldwide.[6]

Once quarantine regulations were strictly enforced, residents of nursing homes were isolated from each other and family members were not allowed to visit. Sadly, many said their last farewells to dying relatives through a bedroom window.

MISSED OPPORTUNITIES

Why would a typically mild infection cause so many more deaths than previous coronaviruses that had higher death rates? The most likely explanation was that because SARS and MERS caused patients to become ill soon after they were infectious, they were quickly out of circulation—before they had a chance to infect too many others. Since those who developed COVID-19 had mild symptoms or none at all, they continued to go to work and socialize, visit elderly relatives in retirement homes and mingle with large crowds in nightclubs or packed sports arenas—all the while, spreading the virus. And so COVID-19 had a wider reach than either SARS or MERS, allowing many more vulnerable people to be exposed and infected.[7]

Public health authorities were slow to pick up on the fact that this asymptomatic spread was largely driving the pandemic. Many researchers expressed frustration at the inaction on the part of authorities as study after study showed that apparently healthy people were major vectors of the disease—spreading the virus while feeling fine themselves. In late May, the Centers for

Disease Control and Prevention (CDC), the US health protection agency that is also a major source of health information for many other countries, finally acknowledged that transmission of the virus by asymptomatic individuals—either silent carriers or those who appeared well but were incubating the disease—was indeed a major problem.[8]

Among residents of long-term care facilities who were particularly at risk of infection and also of having poorer outcomes if they did develop COVID-19, testing for the virus was initially done only on those showing symptoms. But in studies that tested all residents, about 40 per cent tested positive, and of those, about 55 per cent had no symptoms.[9]

It was clear now that the only way to stop the continued spread of the disease was by identifying not just those who were already sick—they were obvious—but also asymptomatic carriers, isolating them and anyone they had recently been in contact with. But this would require mass testing of healthy individuals, along with contact tracing—a Herculean task that few jurisdictions were equipped to undertake.

Since this was a new virus, it would take time for the appropriate tests to be developed and then field-tested for accuracy. After they were validated, laboratory testing capacity would also need to be dramatically increased. At the start, testing and contact tracing seemed pretty haphazard in Canada, with some areas of the country being slower than others to see the need for it. Once tests did become available, some provinces were slower than others to ramp up testing capacity.

There were flip-flops on face masks: at first, the public were told they were unnecessary, but later people were encouraged to wear them when indoors or where social distancing was difficult, like in supermarkets. Eventually, many local governments made them mandatory, especially for travel on public transit and for indoor public spaces. But it was not uncommon to see shoppers entering stores refuse to wear one, even when free masks were offered.

Meanwhile, the virus continued its onward march.

PRE-SYMPTOMATIC AND ASYMPTOMATIC SPREADERS

From the beginning of the pandemic, cruise ships had been seen as ideal breeding grounds for infection. Outbreaks of another virus that caused diarrhea and vomiting—the Norwalk virus— were not uncommon reasons for ships to have to return to port. But Norwalk was a relatively mild gastrointestinal virus that resolved in a few days with little more than supportive care—rest and rehydration.

In early March, the Public Health Agency of Canada recommended against all cruise ship travel due to the risk of COVID-19. Large cruise liners were barred from Canadian waters. "The virus can spread quickly on cruise ships due to the close contact between passengers," said chief public health officer Dr. Theresa Tam as she introduced the new restrictions.

A small ship with 128 passengers and ninety-eight crew members on board left port for a twenty-one-day cruise on March 15,

2020. Starting in Argentina, the ship planned to follow the route taken by the famous Antarctic explorer Sir Ernest Shackleton and his crew between 1915 and 1917. Despite warnings about the potential hazards of cruise travel, it was decided that the trip should go ahead, and the ship set sail as scheduled.[10]

As a precaution, all passengers and crew were carefully screened for the virus before they embarked, and their temperatures were taken. None showed signs of the virus; no one had recently travelled to a known infection hot spot. On board, intensive hygiene precautions and regular temperature and symptom checks were put in place. But despite everyone's best efforts, an unwelcome passenger was stalking the adventurers: COVID-19.

On day eight of the journey, one passenger showed symptoms of the virus and was immediately isolated. The three doctors on board—the ship's physician and two passengers who were doctors—monitored and tried to control the infection. All passengers were confined to their cabins and issued surgical masks. Full personal protective equipment was used by anyone who had contact with symptomatic patients. The crew served meals to cabin doors three times a day, but rooms were not entered for cleaning.

A helicopter dropped rapid testing kits on board, and later, Uruguayan officials took nasal swabs to test for the virus before allowing the ship to finally dock in Montevideo. Writing in the journal *Thorax*, the physicians reported that of the 217 passengers and crew on board, 59 per cent eventually tested positive for COVID-19, among them some who had tested negative using the initial rapid testing. Of those who finally tested positive, sixteen (12.5 per cent) developed fever and mild symptoms. Another eight (6.25 per cent) had to be evacuated to hospital, and four of them (3.1 per cent) ended up in critical care. One unfortunately died—putting the fatality rate at a low 0.8 per cent. But 35 per cent of those who tested positive never developed any symptoms at all.

This story is a textbook example of the epidemiology of COVID-19 infection—the study of how often diseases occur in different groups of people and why. Since the cruise ship and its passengers had no outside human contact for the twenty-eight days they were at sea, this accidental experiment provides solid evidence of how COVID-19 spreads in a totally closed environment. What it couldn't tell us was what the rate of serious illness and death would be if those asymptomatic carriers had hugged their grannies, mixed with friends or relatives undergoing cancer treatment or were in close contact with any of the many other vulnerable groups among the general public—groups that had yet to be identified.

Because of the potential for spread of COVID-19 from those showing no symptoms, strict new rules for social distancing were introduced in most countries, often carrying hefty fines for those who broke them. Everyone was asked to stay at home whenever possible, and if they had to be around other people, to keep at least two metres (or six feet) away from others and wear a mask. In Ireland, for example, the Gardaí (the national police) were given new powers to fine, arrest or even imprison anyone caught travelling more than five kilometres from their own home.

INDIVIDUAL LIBERTY OR THE COMMON GOOD?

One of the most famous cases of asymptomatic disease transmission involves an Irish woman, Mary Mallon, who was working as a cook in New York in the early 1900s. Mary had emigrated from Ireland when she was fifteen and lived with relatives until she started work, first as a housemaid, then as a cook. She apparently changed employment frequently, moving from one wealthy family to another. And wherever Mary worked, people in that household became ill with a bacterial infection caused by *Salmonella typhi*, commonly known as typhoid fever.

Typhoid fever was spread through contaminated food and water or through close contact with someone who was infected. It is thought that Mary was probably born with the disease, since her mother had had typhoid fever while she was pregnant. In New York, the disease was seen mainly in poor inner-city neighbourhoods with high population densities and poor sanitation. But Mary was working in wealthy households, and these were not considered to be at risk for the disease.

Eventually, the link between Mary's presence in a home and the development of typhoid fever in its occupants became clear and "Typhoid Mary," as she was dubbed by the press, was confirmed as the unwitting spreader of the disease. But Mary refused to accept that she was the cause of illness in others, since she felt perfectly well herself. She constantly dodged efforts to restrain her and to prevent her from working. However, over the next twenty-six years, public health authorities hunted her down and forced her into extended periods of quarantine. She died alone and without friends, still quarantined, in 1938.[11]

If historical accounts are accurate, Mary's treatment at the hands of public health authorities was harsh and arrogant, since they apparently failed to explain to her how she was spreading disease and why she needed to be isolated. It probably didn't help, either, that the people she appeared to be infecting were not the poor, but the rich and influential. However, with a 10 per cent mortality rate, the fear of typhoid fever was very real. Effective treatment did not exist at the time, and antibiotics would not become available until 1948—too late for Mary or her victims.

The case stands today as an example of how the moral and legal rights of an individual could be overridden by the need to protect the majority. Mary's incarceration was seen as a necessary sacrifice to the common good—a concept at the core of public health principles today.

OTHER PANDEMICS

In the last hundred years, we have experienced four influenza pandemics as a result of the emergence of new viruses to which populations have no acquired immunity: the H1N1 Spanish flu of 1918–19, the Asian flu of 1957, the Hong Kong flu in 1968, and the swine flu in 2009. The most destructive of all of these was undoubtedly the Spanish flu pandemic of 1918–19.

It started as mild winter flu, no different from any other

seasonal flu. Over the summer months it died down, only to re-emerge towards the end of summer in a much deadlier form. The Spanish flu is estimated to have killed between fifty and one hundred million people worldwide and is the worst pandemic on record. A third wave—less devastating than the second, which had been responsible for most of the fatalities—occurred during the winter and spring of 1919, with the pandemic subsiding in the summer of 1919.

Although called the Spanish flu, there is no evidence the outbreak actually began in Spain. During the First World War (WWI), information on deaths and infections was strictly censored in Europe for fear of demoralizing the troops or giving solace to the enemy. However, Spain was a neutral country and the press there could freely report on the devastating toll the virus was taking. As the only European country to admit it had a problem, Spain therefore looked as if it was the only country suffering. But the pandemic probably started in America and was brought to Europe by American soldiers going to the battlefront to fight in WWI.[12]

While most strains of flu cause the most serious disease in those with lower immunity such as the elderly, the very young or those with pre-existing serious health conditions, the Spanish flu was different, tending to kill healthy adults in the prime of their lives. Most died because of the development of a secondary lung infection, probably bacterial, leading to pneumonia.

Although the exact reason for the vulnerability of younger adults was unclear, it is now believed to be due to the unique ability of the virus to induce a "cytokine storm"—an excessive and uncontrolled overreaction of the immune system that is frequently fatal. This might explain why the disease was more deadly in those with more robust immune responses than in those with weaker immune systems.[13] (We'll talk more about the cytokine storm in later chapters.)

The Spanish flu was brought to Canada by troops returning from Europe at the end of WWI, and it made its way into most communities, where it swept away great swaths of the population, especially in Labrador and Quebec and on First Nations reserves. By 1919 it had caused the death of an estimated fifty-five thousand Canadians, most between the ages of twenty and forty years. It also brought social and economic disruption: families lost their main breadwinner; employers were left without workers. Children became orphans.

Hospital wards, and the nurses and doctors who staffed them, were overwhelmed and volunteers had to organize makeshift treatment centres in schools and hotels. Provinces enacted laws enforcing quarantine. Schools, churches and theatres were shut down. People were advised to avoid shaking hands and to stay indoors, libraries stopped lending books, and new sanitary regulations were introduced. Spitting, a habit that was common at the time, was banned and people were ordered to wear masks in public.

As would happen a hundred years later during the COVID-19 pandemic, the public did not always cooperate, and in many countries arguments raged about whether or not the restrictions imposed on everyday life were economically or socially acceptable. The wearing of face masks was particularly contentious and not everyone would use them. During the Spanish flu pandemic, even front-line workers—doctors and nurses—were sometimes non-compliant.

"When it has been nearly impossible to force the orderlies or even some of the physicians and nurses to wear their masks as prescribed, it is difficult to see how a general measure of this nature could be enforced in the community at large," wrote Dr. Warren T. Vaughan in a 1921 review of the pandemic.[14]

With no known treatments, doctors resorted to prescribing anything they thought might ease symptoms, including very large doses of Aspirin to bring down fever. Anything up to thirty grains—almost two thousand milligrams—was given, and it is believed that some of the deaths attributed to influenza may actually have been due to Aspirin overdose. Doctors thought it was imperative for recovery that patients not be constipated and that bowels "must be kept open." So, liberal amounts of mercurous chloride, one side effect of which was diarrhea, were prescribed to prevent constipation.

Mercurous chloride was extremely toxic. Its more common use was in photography and as a wood preservative. Medically, it had been used to treat syphilis, but because it caused mercury poisoning and was highly damaging to mucous membranes, its use was eventually discontinued. Strychnine, one of the most potent poisons known, was sometimes injected into patients as a stimulant, and the anti-malarial drug quinine hydrochloride was recommended, although there was little evidence it was useful.

Many of the older doctors favoured brandy or whisky in large doses. Soldiers were given rum as a preventative, and in France and elsewhere in Europe, champagne was prescribed, presumably for those who could afford it. Alcohol had a good deal to recommend it, wryly commented one young doctor in Dublin, as even if it didn't cure the disease, patients "would have a merry spin to paradise."[15]

The shambolic response to the 1918–19 pandemic did result in major improvements in public health. In Canada, it prompted the establishment of the federal Department of Health. However, as we battled COVID-19 in 2020, the social, economic and medical problems faced both in Canada and elsewhere didn't seem to have changed much. Even with a greater understanding of immunity and viruses than medicine had in the 1900s, our ability to prevent, detect and treat viral infections in the twenty-first century still seemed rudimentary and public health responses tardy and disorganized.

While progress clearly had been made in controlling infection, and the highly trained doctors and nurses who work heroically round the clock in intensive care units (ICUs) undoubtedly saved many lives, the high infection and mortality rates from COVID-19 nonetheless suggest that in many respects, we have not made much progress in a century of fighting pandemics.

The battle against viruses has not been won.

CHAPTER TWO

The Trouble with Viruses

If it is a terrifying thought that life is at the mercy of the multiplication of these minute bodies [microbes], it is a consoling hope that Science will not always remain powerless before such enemies. —Louis Pasteur (1822–1895)[1]

Long before microbes could be visualized, scholars speculated about their existence and their ability to make people sick. Roman scholar Marcus Terentius Varro (116–27 BC) cautioned against living near swamps. "There are bred certain minute creatures that cannot be seen by the eyes, which float in the air and enter the body through the mouth and nose and there cause serious diseases," he warned.[2] In the sixteenth century, Italian physician and poet Girolamo Fracastoro (1476–1553) proposed that epidemics were caused by "seed-like entities" transmitting disease from person to person, or even over long distances without any person-to-person contact at all. But it wasn't until the invention of the light microscope in the late sixteenth century that these so-far-invisible causes of illness could actually be seen.

The German Jesuit scholar Athanasius Kircher (1601–1680) wrote of his astonishment at discovering innumerable creeping "animalcules" in various foods as he explored the hidden world of microbial life under the newly invented microscope. "Who would believe that vinegar and milk abound with an innumerable multitude of worms," he wrote in 1646.

The "worms" that Kircher observed were in fact bacteria. Viruses, many times smaller than most bacteria, could not be visualized using these early primitive instruments, and it would take the invention of the more powerful electron microscope in the early 1930s before viruses could be examined in detail and the science of virology could begin in earnest.

VIRAL AND BACTERIAL INFECTIONS: SIMILAR BUT DIFFERENT

Bacterial and viral infections frequently cause similar symptoms— coughing and sneezing, fevers, pneumonia, vomiting and diarrhea. However, they differ from each other in important ways—ways that have profound implications for the way each type of microorganism will behave, the health risks they pose and the tools that can be used to prevent and treat the diseases they cause.

Bacteria are living cells, not unlike the cells that make up the human body. Just like our cells, they have an outer retaining wall that provides shape and a boundary to keep internal contents from leaking out. If this wall is breached, the bacterium can't survive. Inside the cell are two large molecules: deoxyribonucleic acid (DNA) and ribonucleic acid (RNA). Together, these two molecules are the basic building blocks of life, containing all the genetic information needed for a bacterium to generate its own energy and to reproduce and make more bacteria.

Because they possess both DNA and RNA, bacteria can live independently, and they have adapted successfully to live just about anywhere. Bacteria have been found at the bottom of deep oceans, in the boiling lava of volcanoes, and even flourishing in radioactive waste. Recently, researchers retrieved mud from below the sea floor in the South Pacific calculated to have settled during the age of the dinosaurs. In the mud were bacteria estimated to be one hundred million years old. With little or no nutrition and minimal oxygen, the bacteria had quietly survived. When supplied with more oxygen and nutrients in the laboratory, they revived, multiplying in number fourfold in a couple of months.[3] "Maintaining full physiological capability for 100 million years in starving isolation is an impressive feat," said oceanographer Steven D'Hondt, one of the researchers involved.

Unlike bacteria, viruses cannot normally survive on their own. This is because the genetic material they contain is composed of either RNA *or* DNA—never both. Since RNA and DNA are both needed for energy generation and reproduction, viruses can have no independent life. To cause infection, they must invade the cell of another organism (the host) and exploit that cell's energy and reproductive capability to create their offspring.

Viruses are therefore sometimes referred to as "parasites," since the definition of a parasite is an organism that survives by living off another organism. But most scientists do not consider viruses to be truly alive, like parasites, but simply non-functional fragments of genetic information, lurking in the environment and generally causing no harm. No harm, that is, until they manage to get inside a living cell.

RNA AND DNA VIRUSES

Mutations—small changes in the structure of genes that can be inherited by future generations—are the building blocks of evolution. Mutations are chance events and do not always benefit viruses. Some, for example, may cause fewer viral offspring to be generated, resulting in these viruses disappearing over time. But the more a virus can mutate, the more likely it is that it will acquire a mutation that increases its infection potential.

DNA viruses possess the ability to detect mutations that may have occurred in their genetic material and repair the errors. Herpesviruses and human papillomavirus (HPV) implicated in cervical cancer are examples of DNA viruses. RNA viruses lack genetic repair mechanisms and therefore evolve more rapidly. Without the ability to repair the errors that frequently occur during replication, RNA viruses are less stable and it is more likely that sooner or later they will acquire a mutation that confers a greater capacity to infect and spread. This is one reason why scientists find it so hard to make vaccines directed against RNA viruses, as they're chasing a constantly moving target.

Coronaviruses are RNA viruses, but with a bit of a twist: they are DNA-virus wannabes. Compared to other RNA viruses, like those that cause seasonal influenza, the genetic material of coronaviruses is more complex and carries instructions that allow them to utilize the host cell's DNA repair mechanisms.[4] Coronaviruses like SARS and COVID-19 are therefore more stable and less likely than other RNA viruses to develop unfavourable mutations that could lead to their demise. They will mutate, but not at the same breathtaking rate of flu viruses.

Strictly speaking, the term "virus" is used for a viral particle that is already inside a cell, initiating infection. When a fully intact virus is outside a cell—lying on the ground or on a doorknob, for instance—it is called a "virion." The virion is the vector—the form that allows transmission of infection and delivers its DNA or RNA to a host cell. However, for the purpose of simplicity, both phases are popularly referred to as "the virus."

Viruses are usually inactivated rapidly on household surfaces, and few remain functional and able to infect for more than a few hours or days. One exception was found when French researchers dug thirty metres under the permafrost in the Siberian tundra. A giant virus—as large as a bacterium—was discovered that had been kept frozen for an estimated thirty thousand years. They named it *Pithovirus sibericum*. Back in the laboratory, the researchers found that the virus could be coaxed into invading cells and causing infection. Fortunately, it only infected tiny unicellular life forms called "amoebas," and posed no threat to humans.[5]

But with rising global warming and the rapid melting of the permafrost, scientists are beginning to wonder whether other ancient viruses might not be liberated from their frozen tombs, and if some of these might not present a threat to animal or human health.

HOW DO BACTERIA CAUSE INFECTIONS?

Historically, bacterial diseases like tuberculosis, typhoid fever and cholera have been major causes of illness and death. Spread through food or water contaminated with feces, or through the air by contact with an infected individual, these diseases were mostly brought under control in developed countries with the establishment of clean water supplies, better housing and the development of antibiotics and vaccines. In economically disadvantaged parts of the world, where conditions of overcrowding and poor sanitation are still common, it's a different matter, and in parts of Africa, China and India, living conditions provide the ideal breeding ground for outbreaks of diseases that are considered a thing of the past in more affluent countries.[6]

Like viruses, bacteria have caused pandemics. Bubonic plague, also known as the Black Death, is caused by the bacterium *Yersinia pestis*. Transmitted by flea bites or contact with contaminated tissues, bubonic plague decimated the population of Europe during the fourteenth century, and successive waves of the infection occurred in Europe, Africa and the Middle East until the end of the nineteenth century. It is still around today—mainly in rural parts of Africa, but it also occasionally crops up in the southwestern United States, where about ten to twenty people become infected each year.

EVERYWHERE YOU LOOK

Viruses are everywhere. They are the most numerous disease-causing organisms on earth. Our oceans teem with them. They are present in dry, sandy deserts. They lurk in the dusty corners of our homes and offices, and are even present in outer space.[7]

Some scientists believe we owe our very existence to viruses, that they provided the molecular raw materials that eventually organized themselves into living cells. Once cellular life was established, so the theory goes, viruses then became the drivers of genetic mutations that led to the evolution and diversification of life on earth, and to the creation of the vast number of plant and animal species that would eventually populate our world.[8]

However, another line of evidence suggests that viruses and bacteria both evolved from a common ancestor—a self-replicating cell that lived around 3.4 billion years ago, when life first emerged on earth. Over time, bacteria became increasingly complex and retained the necessary genes to generate energy and to reproduce. Meanwhile, viruses became simpler—ditching genes they found they could do without, and retaining just enough genetic material to allow them to invade living cells and cunningly persuade those cells to abandon their usual function and instead produce new generations of viruses.[9]

Viruses are seasoned travellers. When heavy winds whip up oceans, they create aerosols, and these aerosols contain viral particles. The aerosols can then get swept up into the troposphere—the layer of the atmosphere closest to earth. Dust storms in dry and arid areas of the world can also launch microbe-laden particles into the troposphere. Strong winds can then carry viruses for thousands of kilometres before they drop back down to earth, deposited either by rain or by direct fallout during dry, calm weather.

Recently, Spanish and Canadian researchers were able to show that even in pristine environments, viruses are showering down on us at an unbelievable rate. "Every day, more than 800 million viruses are deposited per square metre—that's 25 viruses for each person in Canada," says Curtis Suttle from the University of British Columbia, who was involved in the study.[10] Scientists still can't yet say whether any of these microorganisms cause disease. However, some believe that aerosolized influenza viruses swept high into the troposphere, together with the extreme seasonal changes in weather patterns that occur at that altitude, might explain simultaneous outbreaks of flu in widely separated parts of the globe.[11]

HOW VIRUSES INFECT

As with their bacterial counterparts, viral infections generally begin with the virus being inhaled or swallowed. This allows not only for lung and respiratory tract infections to take hold, but also gastrointestinal infections when virus-containing saliva is swallowed. Eyes and breaks in the skin are also potential portals of entry—in fact, any part of the host that is exposed to the external environment is vulnerable.

Before viruses can infect, they must first find an entry point or receptor—a molecular structure on the surface of a potential host's cells to which they can attach. Acting like a key inserted into a lock (and providing it finds a lock that it fits), a virus can then enter the host cell. Some viruses have a fatty outer coating similar to the fatty outside membrane of all mammalian cells. The coronavirus that causes COVID-19 is one of these. These "enveloped viruses" can manufacture special proteins that allow them to fuse with the host cell's membrane and then slip effortlessly inside.

The inner layer of the gastrointestinal tract—the mucosa—is a barrier that needs to be intact to prevent potentially infective microbes and toxins from gaining access to the blood and, through the blood, circulate to other organs. Many viruses, including the virus causing COVID-19, can degrade this gut-blood barrier.[12] Then the virus spreads easily to other organs, leading to their structural damage and progressive loss of function. If this continues unchecked, one or more organs may stop functioning, leading to a frequently fatal condition called multi-organ failure.[13]

STOMACH ACID AND INFECTION

Our secret weapon against gastrointestinal infection is the acid secreted by the stomach, which is an essential part of normal digestion. Most living creatures, including fish, reptiles, birds and mammals, produce stomach acid, suggesting that stomach acid plays a conserved and very basic role in physiology. Gastric acid can kill bacteria and inactivate viruses. Apart from handicapping potentially infective microbes, gastric acid is also needed for the digestion of protein and the absorption of minerals like calcium, iron and zinc. As we get older, low stomach acid becomes more common, leading to mineral deficiencies and improper protein digestion.[14] It also increases the likelihood of gastrointestinal infection.

The good news is that coronaviruses don't seem to survive stomach acid very well, and normal gastric acids levels may therefore reduce the risk of gastrointestinal infection. However, many people take powerful antacid drugs called proton pump inhibitors (PPIs) to treat symptoms of heartburn. These highly efficient drugs are designed to continuously neutralize gastric acid—all day and all night. As might be expected, the frequent use of PPIs is known to increase the risk of many serious infections, not only in the gastrointestinal tract, but also in the lungs.[15]

At Cedars-Sinai Medical Center in Los Angeles, doctors wondered if testing positive for COVID-19 was more common in those taking antacid drugs, and they found that common PPI drugs like omeprazole (Losec), esomeprazole (Nexium) and pantoprazole (Pantoloc) doubled the risk of COVID-19 infection when used once a day, and more than tripled the risk if used twice a day. Other types of antacids, like the H_2-receptor antagonists ranitidine and cimetidine, which don't totally suppress gastric acid, did not seem to increase the risk of infection.[16]

BECOMING VIRAL FACTORIES

Once inside a cell, a virus reprograms the host's genes to mass-produce copies of itself. Eventually, when enough copies accumulate, the cell bursts open, liberating numerous newly generated viruses that are now free to infect other cells or other individuals. But the release of new viruses kills the host cell, causing damage to host tissues. This tissue destruction during infection is one reason why unchecked viral infections make us so sick and can cause lasting organ damage.

Enveloped viruses like coronaviruses can also exit the host cell by budding out through the host's cell wall. As they do so they scoop up some of the host cell's membrane to make a membrane of their own. This borrowed overcoat now acts as a disguise, tricking the host's immune system into believing the virus is not a foreign invader at all, but one of the host's own cells. And so the virus escapes detection. This exit strategy doesn't immediately kill the host cell, but weakens it, and it too eventually will die.

Since up to a million newborn viruses may be released by one infected cell, it's easy to see how one solitary viral particle can be enough to cause extensive infection.[17]

SLEEPERS AND KEEPERS

Some viruses are sleeper viruses. Instead of causing infection right away, they simply insert their genetic instructions into the host's genes and wait. Then, as the host cell reproduces, the virus's genetic instructions get copied, too. Many new generations of cells, each of them carrying rogue viral information, may be produced by the host without causing symptoms. Then, at some later date, something—stress, for example—triggers the virus to wake up and take over the cell, forcing it to begin producing viruses. And infection begins.

The HIV/AIDS virus is a classic example of a sleeper virus. A person may carry it for years, showing no symptoms. But while they may not themselves feel sick, they can pass the virus on to others.[18] At present, there is no cure for HIV/AIDS, but it can be held permanently in check with drugs that stop the virus from replicating. These drugs keep the virus at undetectable levels—levels at which it cannot be transmitted to infect someone else. But the drugs must be taken permanently for the virus to remain under control.

Many viruses become latent in host tissue after an infection has been controlled, but can reactivate later. Most of these viruses belong to the herpes group of viruses, and include herpes simplex, which causes typical blistering cold sores on the lips or genitals, and Epstein-Barr virus—a cause of mononucleosis, sometimes called the "kissing disease" because it is passed on through saliva. Herpesviruses are the most prevalent infectious agents known to exist. By adolescence, nearly everyone is infected with one or multiple herpesviruses, and at any given time it is estimated that they account for between thirty-five and forty billion human infections worldwide.[19]

PERMANENT RESIDENTS

Herpesviruses take up lifetime residency in nerve endings and, in contrast to the AIDS virus, are not asleep at all. Instead, an intense interaction is going on between the herpesvirus and the host's immune system. In healthy individuals, this interaction produces a large pool of immune cells capable of controlling the herpes infection. Like guards in a jailhouse, the immune cells keep the virus prisoner, limiting its activity so it causes no symptoms.

This constant low-level activation of immune cells by herpesviruses not only controls the herpes infection, it has several other benefits, one of which is to prevent allergies.[20] Another is to keep cells called natural killer cells (NK cells) active and alert. NK cells are immune cells that scout out and kill virally infected cells, and they can also detect and control early signs of cancer.[21]

However, with latent viruses, recurrence of an active infection is always just around the corner, especially if we need to take medications that suppress immunity, like steroids or chemotherapy drugs. Moreover, many different types of stress suppress immunity and can trigger the re-emergence of herpes infections, including the stress of infection due to other viruses, or physical stress like trauma. Psychological stress, especially if prolonged, is a major case of reactivation.[22]

Exposure to intense sunlight can also stimulate a resurgence of symptoms,[23] as anyone who has had a sunshine vacation spoiled by a sudden outbreak of cold sores can confirm. This is because the UV rays damage and ultimately kill the immune cells assigned to control the virus.[24] Sunscreen applied regularly to the lips while in the sun will protect against this damage and limit outbreaks.[25]

BREAKING AND ENTERING

Viral receptors are not present on cells simply to satisfy the requirements of the virus; they are vitally important for the host. Unfortunately, the binding of a virus to the host receptor disrupts its normal function, often with predictable consequences. For example, several different families of viruses, including herpesviruses, can use a cell-surface molecule called the transferrin receptor as an entry point. One of the transferrin receptor's normal roles is to absorb iron and then distribute it where it is needed—particularly to the bone marrow, where new red cells are made. Chronic herpes infection interferes with this function and, not unexpectedly, can lead to anemia.[26]

To invade cells, coronaviruses that cause SARS and COVID-19 exploit a receptor called the angiotensin-converting enzyme 2 (ACE2) receptor. ACE2 receptors are plentiful on the mucous membranes of the nose, throat and lungs, and are also present in heart, intestine, kidney and liver tissue. The viruses latch onto the ACE2 receptor using spike-like proteins on their outer coat. In doing so, they block the normal function of ACE2 receptors. However, functional ACE2 receptors are vital to the health of the host. They help regulate blood pressure and control the utilization of minerals by the body. They also dampen down inflammation and protect lungs from severe injury.

The soft, spongy tissue of the lungs is made up of millions of tiny air sacs called alveoli. It is in these air sacs that gas exchange takes place—where the oxygen we breathe in diffuses into the blood for circulation, and where carbon dioxide, a toxic waste product of metabolism, leaves the blood and enters the lungs, to be removed when we breathe out. ACE2 receptors are abundant in alveoli.

One outcome of spike proteins binding to ACE2 receptors is uncontrolled inflammation. Another is that cells stop secreting a lung-protective fluid called surfactant. Without normal surfactant, the alveoli collapse like so many deflated balloons. As a consequence, the passage of oxygen into the blood is drastically reduced and the passage of carbon dioxide out of the blood and into the lungs for disposal also stops.[27]

This explains why emergency room doctors were at first mystified by COVID-19 patients arriving at hospitals with dangerously low blood oxygen levels and X-ray evidence of pneumonia, but with no apparent difficulty breathing, since it is the accumulation of carbon dioxide in the lungs that usually causes breathing difficulties. However, over time, the lungs of these patients were increasingly damaged by inflammation, and then breathing became so difficult that some patients required not just oxygen to survive, but also the mechanical help of a ventilator.

VIRUSES ARE BAD NEWS

British immunologist Sir Peter Medawar (1915–1987), winner of the Nobel Prize in Physiology or Medicine in 1960, once famously quipped, "A virus is a piece of bad news wrapped in protein." And bad news many of them are. However, the diseases they cause run the gamut from severe, life-threatening infections like HIV/AIDS or Ebola, to common childhood illnesses like measles and mumps, to everyday nuisances like the common cold or seasonal flu.

Smallpox, caused by the variola virus, once ravaged Europe and the Old World, killing 30 per cent of those who got it and blinding or disfiguring many more. The symptoms of smallpox include many small blisters on the face, arms and body, which fill up with pus. When these heal, they leave characteristic pitting scars or "pockmarks." Smallpox was brought to the Americas by Spanish and Portuguese explorers in the sixteenth century, where it decimated Indigenous populations who had no natural immunity to it. After the development of effective vaccines, we no longer had to worry about smallpox, and in 1980 the World Health Assembly triumphantly announced that smallpox had been eradicated. The world was now free of the virus.

Although it sounds as if it is related to smallpox, chickenpox is caused by a different virus, the varicella-zoster virus, and is substantially less deadly. Chickenpox used to be a common illness, especially in children. Before the development of the chickenpox vaccine, it made about four million people sick every year and sent thousands to hospital. Since the introduction of vaccination in Canada at the beginning of the twenty-first century, chickenpox is much rarer but hasn't been completely eradicated.

Chickenpox is a herpesvirus, so after chickenpox infection, the virus never completely clears from the system but remains latent in nerve endings, where it is kept in check by cells of the immune system. Years later, if immunity is compromised by illness or stress, the virus can reactivate as shingles, a non-infective but painful, blistery skin rash. In some people, shingles leads to intense neurological pain at the site of the eruption that can last for months or even years. Although it is most common in people who have had active chickenpox infection, it occasionally occurs after chickenpox vaccination.[28]

Most of us are familiar with measles, mumps and rubella, three common childhood viral illnesses. A vaccine against all three—the MMR vaccine—was introduced in Canada in 1983 and is now routinely given to all infants. The MMR vaccine is made up of viruses that have been treated to make them weaker—too weak to cause an infection, but still able to induce the body to produce an immune response that protects against future exposure to these common viruses.

TREATING BACTERIAL INFECTIONS

Bacterial infections caused potentially devastating diseases until well into the twentieth century. Then, a happy accident in 1928 led to the development of the first antibiotic. Returning from holiday, bacteriologist Alexander Fleming noticed that one of the petri dishes in which he had been growing staphylococcus bacteria was contaminated with a mould or fungus. To his surprise, the fungus appeared to be severely suppressing the growth of the bacteria.

The contaminating fungus was identified as *Penicillium notatum*, and the bacteria-killing molecule it produced was named "penicillin." Fleming published his findings in 1929,[29] but it was not until the early 1940s that collaborative efforts between governments, industry and British and American scientists led to enough penicillin being manufactured to carry out large-scale testing in human subjects.

Antibiotics deal with infection in one of two ways. They may be bacteriostatic—that is, they slow down the growth of bacteria and give the body's own natural defences a chance to kick in and clear up the infection. Or, they may kill a bacterium outright, usually by weakening its ability to manufacture a proper cell wall. The latter is the way penicillin works. Penicillin was probably pivotal in winning the Second World War. Prior to its development, thousands of injured soldiers died from infected wounds. But with the introduction of penicillin, once-fatal bacterial infections became treatable, and soldiers lived to fight another day.[30]

By the end of World War II, penicillin was being widely used, not just on battlefields but in hospitals, and had saved so many lives that it was nicknamed "the wonder drug." Between the 1940s and 1960s—considered the golden age of antibiotic discovery—scientists harvested many new molecules with antibiotic properties, not just from fungi but also from various soil microbes, which pharmaceutical companies developed into lucrative new drugs.

ANTIBIOTICS: VICTIMS OF THEIR OWN SUCCESS?

While some antibiotics attack only a limited range of bacteria, others—called broad spectrum antibiotics—seek and destroy a wide range of unrelated bacteria. The development of this scattergun approach to treating bacterial infection at first seemed invaluable, since the drugs could be used without waiting for the results of laboratory tests to identify exactly which bacteria were causing an infection. But as their use continued, several serious drawbacks emerged.

A world of microbes—many trillions of bacteria, viruses and fungi—colonizes the interior and exterior of our bodies, where they live together in a complex and not yet fully understood dynamic. Now collectively known as "the microbiome," these tiny guests are part of our natural defences against parasites and other pathogens. Bacteria are overwhelmingly the most numerous organisms in the microbiome, and many play essential roles not only in gut health, but also in the digestion and metabolism of food and in weight control.[31]

Many scientists consider the microbiome almost as a separate organ since it produces a myriad of health-promoting molecules, some of which are actually critical for our own survival. For example, bacteria in a healthy microbiome can contribute to our nutrition by producing certain essential vitamins—the B vitamins and vitamin K. The microbiome also plays a critical role in regulating immunity, essentially training an army of immune cells to recognize unwelcome invaders and respond appropriately to infection.[32]

As we learn more about the microbiome, we can see that the enthusiastic and liberal use of antibiotics in the latter part of the twentieth century, especially broad spectrum antibiotics, has led to the indiscriminate killing of these protective bacteria. A number of health conditions, including cancer, obesity and bowel disorders like ulcerative colitis and Crohn's disease, have been linked to frequent antibiotic use.[33] Recently, researchers found that a healthy microbiome in the nose and throat can protect against seasonal influenza.[34] It is conceivable that disturbance of the respiratory microbiome by antibiotics might therefore increase susceptibility to other respiratory viruses like coronaviruses.

The good news is that after stopping antibiotics, our microbiomes can return to normal. Well, almost. When a team of researchers in Denmark gave young, healthy men three antibiotics for four days, they found virtually complete eradication of bacteria in their intestines. Over the next six months, they observed a gradual recovery and a return of most normal bacterial species, but a few new and potentially undesirable bacteria had also taken up residence, the long-term consequences of which are unknown.[35]

ANTIBIOTIC RESISTANCE

Another worrying problem that is emerging from the unrestrained use of antibiotics is the development of antibiotic resistance. Occasionally, among all the bacteria causing an infection, one may adapt to survive treatment. This "resistant" bacterium can now multiply and create offspring that are no longer sensitive to antibiotics. And the more frequent the use of antibiotics, the more likely it is that resistant bacteria will develop and existing antibiotic drugs will become ineffective.[36] Antibiotic resistance is now a global health crisis due to the overuse of antibiotics in humans and in animals.[37]

In the early days of the COVID-19 crisis, many patients were at first given antibiotics because of their symptoms—cough, fever and X-ray evidence of lung infection, symptoms that are hallmarks of bacterial pneumonia. While secondary bacterial infections may develop occasionally during viral infections, including during COVID-19 infection, for the most part antibiotic use is ineffective, since antibiotics have no impact on viral diseases.

The early overuse of antibiotics was eventually halted, but there remains lingering concern that the inappropriate use of antibiotics in COVID-19 patients may have exacerbated antibiotic resistance, already considered a pandemic in its own right. "The COVID-19 pandemic has led to an increased use of antibiotics, which ultimately will lead to higher bacterial resistance rates that will impact the burden of disease and deaths during the pandemic and beyond," warned Tedros Adhanom Ghebreyesus, director general of the WHO.

KILLING THE VIRUS WITHOUT
KILLING THE HOST

Compared to treating bacterial infections, the treatment of viral infections is much more challenging. All bacteria have a similar cell wall, so drugs that damage this wall or interfere with its assembly will effectively kill them. Bacterial cells have many features that are different from human cells, and these differences can be exploited to make antibacterial drugs. For example, the cell walls of bacteria contain large molecules called "peptidoglycans," which are not present on human or other mammalian cells. Drugs designed to target this molecule will therefore kill the offending bacterium while causing minimal collateral damage to host cells.

In contrast, viruses cause infection only when they are inside living cells, so any assault on a virus will also be an assault on the host. Unlike antibiotics, antiviral drugs do not destroy viruses, which are not technically alive in the first place, and so can't be killed. Instead, antiviral drugs block viruses from replicating, preventing the virus increasing in numbers to a point where the body's natural antiviral defences are overwhelmed. But the replication machinery of the virus is also needed by host cells, so any drug that targets viral replication is potentially toxic to the host.

Successful antiviral drugs target some process or molecular structure unique to the virus that is not present on human tissue. While all bacteria have many molecular features in common, viruses are extremely diverse. This makes it difficult to find a target that is common to a wide range of viruses, which would allow for the creation of broad spectrum antiviral drugs to be created that are effective, yet don't cause more harm than good. This difficulty is one reason why viral infections, by their very nature, present so much more of a problem to treat successfully than bacterial infections.

DISARMING THE VIRUS

One approach to controlling viral infection without harming the host is to find a way to block a virus from entering a cell. As we have seen, COVID-19 uses the spike proteins on its surface to lock onto ACE2 receptors. Any molecule that could bind to the spike protein would potentially neutralize the virus, blocking it from binding to ACE2 receptors. In the next chapter, we will see how the immune system can do this, producing neutralizing antibodies that bind to the spike protein and thwart infection.

But binding to ACE2 receptors alone isn't enough for infection to begin; for the genetic viral material to enter a cell, the spike protein must be left behind. To do this, the virus co-opts a protein-cutting enzyme called furin—an enzyme essential to the normal metabolism of the host cell—to split the spike protein open, allowing the virus to enter. Any molecule that could block these molecular scissors could therefore limit the spread of the virus.[38] Furin is present in most tissues and is particularly rich in the lungs. The ability of COVID-19 to co-opt the host cells' furin is thought to be one reason COVID-19 is more pathogenic and spreads more easily throughout the body than other coronaviruses.[39]

Several drugs already exist that prevent the splitting of the spike protein. One of them is the much-maligned anti-malarial drug hydroxychloroquine, now no longer authorized for COVID-19 treatment or prevention. The other is the antiviral drug Remdesivir, which has been shown to shorten patients' time in ICU from fifteen days to ten and reduce mortality by 4.8 per cent.[40]

HOW TO BE A SUCCESSFUL VIRUS

Because it can only replicate in a living cell, it isn't in the best interest of a virus to kill its host. So, the most successful virus would be one that was highly contagious, causing only mild-to-moderate symptoms in most people and allowing the host to feel well enough for a period of time after infection to work and socialize. It should be a novel virus, one that no one has experienced before and to which no specific immunity has developed.

To really thrive, the virus should be easily transmitted. Viruses can be spread through contaminated blood or other body fluids, as in HIV/AIDS, or through food or water contaminated with fecal matter from an infected person, as in polio or hepatitis A. Or they can be transmitted by the respiratory route, where coughing or sneezing, singing, talking or even breathing can transfer virus-laden droplets and aerosols from person to person. Of all of the methods of transmission, a successful virus would be well advised to follow the respiratory route.

Viral receptors, needed for the virus to gain access to a cell and begin reproducing, are highly specific to a particular type of virus. So, a successful virus would be one that has evolved to use receptors that are widespread on the host's tissues, especially those of the nose, throat and lungs. And in order to jump from animals to humans—in so-called "zoonotic" diseases—the original animal host must also be well endowed with the same receptors.

If a virus could fulfill all these criteria—be newly mutated to spread from animals to humans; be mildly infective in most people; be spread by the respiratory route and use a receptor to gain entry that is plentiful in the upper respiratory tract—it would indeed be a very successful virus, especially if it were an enveloped virus, one that could cloak itself in the cellular membrane of the host and become invisible to immune detection.

If such a virus were to emerge, international travel for business or pleasure would then ensure its worldwide spread and we would have a pandemic on our hands.

WHAT SCIENTISTS PREDICTED

On November 9, 2017, a meeting was convened at Johns Hopkins University's Center for Health Security in Baltimore, Maryland. At the meeting were national and international scientists, representatives of American and foreign academic institutions, and the US federal government. The meeting's purpose was to explore what was known about the characteristics of microbes that posed the greatest threat to public health. Could a profile be developed of an infectious disease outbreak that was ominous—one that should alert us to its pandemic potential, that could lead to a "sudden, extraordinary, widespread disaster beyond the collective capability of national and international governments and the private sector to control"?[41]

The consensus of that meeting was clear. There were definitive identifiable traits a microbe with the potential for pandemic spread was likely to possess, the scientists warned. Surveillance systems should be on the lookout for any microbe making its first foray into human populations if it fulfilled the following characteristics:

> . . . efficient human-to-human transmissibility, an appreciable case fatality rate, the absence of effective or widely available medical countermeasures, an immunologically naive population, and a respiratory mode of spread. Additionally, the ability to be transmitted during incubation periods, and/or the occurrence of mild illnesses would facilitate spread. Viruses are the most likely class of microorganisms to have this capacity.

The meeting at Johns Hopkins was not intended as an idle academic exercise; rather, it was an attempt to come up with a framework for the surveillance of the infectious disease landscape, so that any agent to emerge anywhere in the world could be recognized early and responded to promptly, and widespread medical, social and economic devastation could be averted.[42]

In 2019, such a virus did emerge and was eventually called SARS-COV2. The illness it caused was known as COVID-19.

CHAPTER THREE

The Immune System Fights Back

Whenever the immune system deals successfully with an infection,
it emerges from the experience stronger and better able to confront
similar threats in the future. Our immune system develops in combat.
—*Andrew Weil, MD (1942–), Professor, University of Arizona
College of Medicine–Tucson*

If we are constantly exposed to viruses and other disease-causing microbes, what prevents us from being constantly sick? Our immune system consists of a network of cells, organs, biomolecules and processes, and is there to protect us. It is working continuously, often silently, to recognize potentially harmful microbes and eliminate them.

When everything is running smoothly, we are completely unaware of our immune system working away in the background. But if the system falters—perhaps because we are stressed and rundown or we've been exposed to a germ we have never encountered before—we become ill. A cold or the flu is a sign your immune system has been overwhelmed by a virus and failed to get the infection under control at its earliest stages.

While each element of the immune system has a distinct role to play, our overall ability to protect ourselves from pathogens depends on the efficient functioning of the entire network.[1]

INNATE VERSUS ACQUIRED IMMUNITY

There are two basic parts to the immune system: the innate immune system and the adaptive or acquired immune response.

Innate immunity consists of physical and chemical barriers to infection as well as specialized cells that seek out and destroy invaders. Because it responds in the same way to all foreign material—bacteria, viruses, abnormal cells like cancer cells, and even non-living materials like dust particles or toxins—it is also known as non-specific immunity. The main cellular components of immunity are white blood cells called leucocytes, and these include several specialized subtypes—lymphocytes, monocytes, neutrophils, macrophages and natural killer cells—all of which have their own special roles to play.

Physical barriers to infection include skin, the tough outer layer of which consists of dry, dead cells that are difficult for pathogens to penetrate. The mucous membranes lining the respiratory, gastrointestinal, urinary and reproductive tracts also provide effective barriers. The mucus they secrete is sticky and traps microbes, blocking them from adhering to cells and infiltrating tissues. Hairs in the respiratory tract oscillate back and forth, sweeping microbes away from epithelial surfaces. Microbes are then expelled by coughing or sneezing.

In addition to physical barriers, body fluids contain chemical substances that create an inhospitable environment for infection. Sweat glands and hair follicles secrete lactic acid, which inhibits microbial growth. Saliva and mucus in the mouth and esophagus contain enzymes that can disable viruses and kill bacteria. Organisms that survive the acidic environment of the stomach face an onslaught of other antimicrobial compounds farther down the gastrointestinal tract. Similarly, tears, ear wax and vaginal secretions all contain protective antimicrobials.

If an organism does make it past these physical and chemical barriers, innate immune cells are primed for immediate response.

FIRST RESPONDERS

In 1882, Russian scientist Élie Metchnikoff (1845–1916) was living in exile in Sicily, having fled Russia during the political upheaval that followed the assassination of Tsar Alexander II. One day, looking down his microscope at cells moving around inside the transparent body of a starfish larva, he found himself wondering if these mobile cells could be the larva's natural defence against intruders.

Collecting some thorns from a tangerine tree in his garden, he inserted one into the body of each tiny creature. If his theory was right, he reasoned, those itinerant cells should begin to congregate around the thorns and try to get rid of them. Next day, he saw that larval cells were indeed clustered around the thorns and attempting to ingest them. Metchnikoff went on to show that similar scavenger cells circulated in human blood, and that these were capable of engulfing and killing micro-organisms—a discovery that earned him a share of the Nobel Prize for Physiology or Medicine in 1908. These predatory cells were later named "phagocytes" (from the Greek: *phagein* = eating + *kytos* = cell).

Phagocytes are the first responders of the innate immune system. Many types of human cells have phagocytic activity. Among the most effective are macrophages and neutrophils. Macrophages begin life in the blood as monocytes and mature into macrophages when they leave the blood and migrate into tissues. Macrophages are particularly active in the lungs, where they free the airways of the daily onslaught of bacteria and other micro-organisms we breathe in, as well as non-living elements like dust particles.

Neutrophils are short-lived white cells that are replenished from the bone marrow in large numbers every day. They remain in the blood until they reach an area of infection or inflammation; then they squeeze out of blood vessels and into the tissue. While neutrophils will engulf any microbe randomly encountered, both macrophages and neutrophils have special homing skills that specifically attract them to sites of infection.

How this homing mechanism works was unclear until the 1990s, when it was discovered that all microbes—viruses, bacteria and fungi—have unique patterns of molecules on their surface that are not present on human cells. Phagocytic cells have receptors called pattern recognition molecules on their cell surfaces, which they use to detect these alien patterns and home in on pathogens.[2] Once phagocytes have made contact with a pathogen, they bind to it, drawing the microbe inside and killing or disabling it so it cannot cause infection.

Some of the best studied pattern recognition molecules are called Toll-like receptors (TLRs). TLRs are plentiful on the surfaces of macrophages and neutrophils.[3] They help phagocytic cells distinguish between tissues that are "self" (that is, healthy cells that belong in the body) and those that are "non-self," like microbes. Using TLRs, phagocytic cells can also recognize and delete "altered self"—host cells that are either damaged, virally infected or have turned cancerous.

Other white cells called natural killer cells (NK-cells) are also first responders. NK-cells kill and eliminate infected or stressed cells, as well as cancer cells. They also release cytokines like interferon, which activates macrophages. In turn, activated macrophages secrete additional interferon and other cytokines, stimulating NK-cells. This cycle of mutual activation enhances the activity of both NK-cells and macrophages, and amplifies innate immune responses. Interferon is critical in preventing the spread of infection in the early stages.[4] However, its release causes many of the symptoms we associate with fighting an infection—chills, fever, body aches and fatigue.

Innate immunity, also known as natural or non-specific immunity, is present from the moment we are born. Over the course of our lifetimes, it won't change very much. But it varies in effectiveness from person to person. Scientists don't quite understand the reason, but think that multiple factors may be involved, some of them genetic and some non-genetic.

Age certainly plays a role. For example, babies born prematurely are more susceptible to viral infections than those born full term, in part due to lower numbers of TLRs on the surface of their immune cells.[5] A similar mechanism seems to be at work in the elderly, who also have fewer TLRs on phagocytic cells, and this may blunt their innate immune responses, making it more difficult for them to control an infection promptly, before it gets out of hand.[6]

HOW FEVERS WORK

As a response to infection, one of the cytokines released by macrophages, interleukin-1, turns up the body's thermostat. The increased body temperature enhances the metabolic activity of immune cells and speeds up innate immune responses.

In the days before antibiotics were available, fevers were sometimes intentionally induced to fight infection. Syphilis and gonorrhea, two sexually transmitted bacterial diseases, were untreatable in the pre-antibiotic era. Although neither infection usually caused a fever, laboratory testing found that both bacteria were killed at higher than normal body temperatures. Patients were therefore deliberately infected with malaria, and the fever that followed was sufficient to eradicate the syphilis or gonorrhea.

Of course, the patients now had malaria, but this could be cured if they were given quinine, an effective and relatively safe treatment. This approach to treating otherwise untreatable infections was considered such a medical breakthrough that in 1927, Julius Wagner-Jauregg, the Austrian neurologist who pioneered the method, was awarded the Nobel Prize in Physiology or Medicine.

Several over-the-counter drugs bring elevated temperatures down into the normal range (a fever is usually defined as a body temperature of 38 degrees Celsius—100.4 degrees Fahrenheit—or higher). They include Aspirin, heavily used during the 1918–19 Spanish flu and still used today, and other anti-inflammatory drugs like acetaminophen and ibuprofen. But should you use them and suppress a fever, or would you get better faster if you let it persist?

One school of thought believes it is better to suppress a fever, arguing that the high energy costs required to sustain a fever are simply too much of a drain on the resources of an already stressed host. Others believe that under most circumstances, a fever will help clear the infection sooner and should not be suppressed. Recently, several randomized controlled trials have lent support to the latter theory, and show that during infection outcomes may be better if the fever is allowed to run its course.[7]

ADAPTIVE OR ACQUIRED IMMUNITY

Whereas the job of innate immunity is to shut down infection as quickly as possible, adaptive immunity is ready to respond in case the innate immune response is inadequate. Adaptive immunity is also known as "acquired immunity" since, depending on which organisms we have been exposed to over the course of our lifetimes, adaptive immune responses develop and change.

Once in contact with an infectious agent, innate immune cells secrete chemical messengers called "cytokines." Cytokines are protein molecules that work either directly on invaders to prevent them from replicating, or indirectly by recruiting more immune cells to join the fight. Interferon is one of the best known of these cytokines. Others include interleukins and tumour necrosis factors.

Some phagocytes will also shift particles from the pathogens they have chewed up back onto their outer surface and present them, like trophies of war, to other cells of the immune system. This, too, is a cue to the adaptive immune system to get busy. The pathogen fragments are called "antigens," and the phagocytic cells that display them on their surface are called "antigen-presenting cells."

The most efficient antigen-presenting cells are dendritic cells, so called because of their unusual shape and many protruding arms or branches (dendrites). Dendritic cells are present in almost all tissues, and are particularly rich in tissues that are in contact with the external environment, including the skin, the lining of the nose and throat, the lungs and the gastrointestinal tract. Dendritic cells are uniquely able to initiate, coordinate and regulate immune responses, and they serve as a bridge between innate and adaptive immunity.

While cytokines are essential players in the response to infection, in excess they can be harmful.[8] The "cytokine storm" seen in the most severely ill COVID-19 patients occurs when there is uncontrolled and excessive release of cytokines. The poor outcomes seen in these patients demonstrates how necessary it is to be able to curb immune responses and prevent them from causing harm.

Ultimately, it is the complex interplay of cytokines and the cells they regulate that drives the body's antimicrobial defences, switching immune responses on when needed, and then off again when their work is done. Over forty molecules have been discovered that have cytokine activity.

A SLOW START

Two types of white blood cells—B lymphocytes and T lymphocytes—are the main players in adaptive immunity. Starting life as stem cells in the bone marrow, those destined to become B cells mature in the bone marrow, while those destined to become T cells migrate to the thymus gland—a small organ located just below the breastbone—to mature. We will revisit the thymus gland later when we consider the role of nutrition in immunity.

The main job of B cells is to secrete antibodies. Antibodies, also known as immunoglobulins, are Y-shaped molecules that bind tightly to the surface of invading pathogens and interfere with a virus's ability to bind to host tissues and complete its invasion of host cells. Antibodies that block the binding of viruses to host cell receptors are called "neutralizing antibodies."

Three types of T cells play different but linked roles in adaptive immunity: cytotoxic T cells, T helper cells and regulatory T cells. Cytotoxic cells directly kill virally infected cells and cancer cells, leaving healthy cells unharmed. As their name suggests, T helper cells assist other immune cells in performing specific functions— triggering antibody secretion by B cells, stimulating macrophages to ingest and destroy microbes, and activating cytotoxic T cells. Regulatory T cells (T regs), previously known as suppressor T cells, help to control the magnitude of the immune response. Like the conductor of an orchestra, they instruct players to ramp up the volume at certain times but play softly at others. Not just essential in fighting infection, T regs are also necessary to prevent the overreaction of the immune system that leads to autoimmune disease or a cytokine storm.[9]

Autoimmune diseases develop when the immune system mistakenly identifies the body's own cells or fragments of damaged tissue as "foreign" and starts attacking healthy tissue.[10] A growing body of research suggests that in some genetically susceptible individuals, unregulated, ramped-up responses to herpes and other common viruses could prompt the development of autoimmune diseases like celiac disease, type 1 diabetes, rheumatoid arthritis or multiple sclerosis.[11]

Through ongoing stimulation of immunity, we generate a near-limitless variety of lymphocytes, each with different receptors on their surfaces, and so there are always a few T and B cells circulating that are capable of recognizing antigens from virtually any infecting pathogen. Once alerted to an invader by an antigen-presenting cell, T and B cells that recognize that antigen become active.

Activated B cells now begin dividing to produce daughter cells, which in turn divide to produce several more generations. This process is called "clonal expansion," as each new generation of cells is a clone or carbon copy of the original cell that responded to the pathogen and can produce neutralizing antibodies that bind to that pathogen to block infection. Clonal expansion amplifies the response to a new threat.

While the innate immune response should be agile and respond quickly to infection, the adaptive response is stronger and long-lasting. But because clonal expansion takes time, the adaptive immune response may take days or even weeks to become fully effective.

FACING THE ENEMY

In the war against infection, think of phagocytic cells like macrophages, neutrophils and dendrites as the foot soldiers, patrolling tissues on the lookout for a security breach. If invaders are encountered, the foot soldiers begin the fight with the weapons they have at hand. At the same time, they send messages (interferon and other cytokines; antigen-presenting cells) to their "squadron leader" to be prepared to provide backup—more troops, with more sophisticated weaponry.

Sometimes, foot soldiers alone can subdue the enemy, and then the damage done to tissues is minimal. Sometimes an entire army may be required, particularly when the number of invaders is high (that is, when there is a high viral load). War is inevitably a violent and messy affair, and the war on viruses is no exception. With many more soldiers appearing on the scene launching missiles and mortar attacks, there is likely to be substantial infrastructure damage. Fires break out (inflammation); buildings (tissues and organs) may be damaged.

An efficient and disciplined army may win the battle without too much local destruction, but a battalion with poor leadership that runs amok and continues random attacks long after the battle is won (as in a cytokine storm) will inflict considerable harm. After the war is over, some damage may be permanent. Certainly, a lot of cleanup and repair will be necessary. The raw material for all that activity can only come from one source: the proteins, fats, vitamins and minerals present in our food, or supplied through nutritional supplements.

We will explore in later chapters how we can support innate immune responses using optimal nutrition to control COVID-19 infection in the earliest stages, to counter overactive inflammatory responses that lead to a cytokine storm, and to support healing and recovery after infection.

REMEMBRANCE OF THINGS PAST

A unique property of the adaptive immune response is that it has memory—it can store information about any microbe it has been exposed to and, if the same microbe is encountered again, quickly spring into action and see it off. Immune memory is stored in subsets of B and T lymphocytes called, appropriately, "memory cells." This time around, there is no delay, and memory cells may remain ready to respond efficiently many years after the first encounter with a pathogen. Generally speaking, memory cells provide lasting protection from the same microbe if it is encountered again—mostly, but not always. For example, if you have had measles, you are probably immune for life. But viruses that cause seasonal flu do not induce long-lasting memory, and we are easily reinfected on repeat exposure.

Vaccination uses the immune system's ability to "remember" so that individuals can develop protection against infectious diseases they have not previously encountered. Vaccination involves a controlled exposure to an altered version of a microbe—or part of a microbe—provoking a mini-infection. The infection is so mild that it causes only minor symptoms or none at all, but it is sufficient to induce memory T and B cells. Vaccination trains the immune system to recognize and respond quickly when exposed to dangerous diseases like polio or measles.

How vaccination was discovered and developed into the science we know today is really the story of smallpox, a disease that has periodically devastated communities since the beginning of recorded history. In eighteenth-century Europe, an estimated

400,000 people died from it annually, and one-third of survivors went blind. Children were especially susceptible. Late in the nineteenth century, 80 per cent of children living in London who contracted smallpox died, while almost 100 per cent of infected children living in Berlin succumbed.[12]

A very early observation was the fact that anyone who survived smallpox infection was safe from reinfection. As far back as the fifth century BC, smallpox survivors were used to nurse smallpox victims because they were the only ones who could do the job safely.[13] One method of prevention—inoculation—appears to have been discovered simultaneously in several different countries faced with smallpox epidemics. The procedure involved taking the contents of a pustule on the skin of a person with active but mild smallpox infection, smearing it on a lancet, and using this to introduce the live virus under the skin of a non-immune person. This approach to dealing with smallpox was called "variolation" (from "variola," or smallpox) and was the earliest form of immunization.

While variolation could protect against smallpox, the practice was risky. Some recipients got smallpox from the inoculum, and between 2 and 3 per cent of these died. Others survived but infected others and became the source of new epidemics. Then a British doctor, Edward Jenner (1749–1823), heard rumours that dairymaids, known for their fine complexions, were protected from smallpox if they had previously been infected with cowpox—a closely related virus that produced a much milder infection and did not cause blindness or disfigure the face.

In May 1796, Jenner used material from a young dairymaid

with fresh cowpox pustules on her hands and arms to inoculate an eight-year-old boy. The boy developed cowpox. After he recovered, Jenner inoculated him with a heavy dose of smallpox. When the boy did not develop smallpox, Jenner saw that this method could provide complete protection against the disease. He called his procedure "vaccination," from the Latin *vacca*, meaning "cow."

Modern-day vaccines have been around since the beginning of the twentieth century and are considered one of the most successful and cost-effective medical interventions in human history.[14] They have been revolutionary in reducing the incidence of viral diseases like polio, measles and chickenpox. More recently, vaccines have been used to prevent common infections like seasonal influenza, hepatitis A and B, and HPV.

HERD IMMUNITY AND COVID-19

Herd immunity is said to exist when the number of people in a community who are immune to a virus—either through vaccination or natural infection—is high enough that the chance of an infected person coming in contact with individuals who are not immune to the disease is greatly reduced. Although an individual may still get infected when good herd immunity exists, the risk of an outbreak is minimized.

Herd immunity is an important concept in vaccinology, since not everyone can be protected by vaccines. Some individuals may be unresponsive to them; others may have allergies to components of a vaccine, or health conditions that make the use of certain vaccines hazardous. To protect vulnerable individuals from COVID-19, the WHO has suggested that 60 to 70 per cent of the population would need to have developed herd immunity.

It has been suggested that instead of trying to prevent coronavirus infection, we should let the virus run amok and allow as many people as possible to get the virus, prompting herd immunity to develop naturally. Essentially, this would mean taking minimal preventive measures. We could avoid school and workplace closures. There would be no lockdowns or shelter-in-place orders, and no requirement for social distancing or wearing masks. According to proponents of this approach, the net benefits might be worth the burden of infection, since all these measures place us under considerable social, psychological and economic stress.

Several countries have considered this approach, including the UK and Sweden. The UK backtracked and imposed a lockdown in the early days of the pandemic, when the strain on the health-care system and the number of deaths attributable to COVID-19 became unacceptable. Sweden decided to let the virus spread among young people, and did not impose lockdowns or close bars or nightclubs. They did take steps to protect the elderly and the medically vulnerable and suggested that people work from home where possible. They limited the size of public gatherings to fifty. But restaurants, gyms, shops, playgrounds and most schools remained open.

The experiment was not widely viewed as a success. Herd immunity sufficient to protect most of the population did not appear to have been achieved during the first wave, and compared to neighbouring countries, Sweden's death toll relative to the size of its population was staggeringly high.[15] Nor did it appear that Sweden gained any economic advantage: the financial downturn, including unemployment, in Sweden was similar to neighbouring countries where stricter public health measures were enforced, while the death rates in those countries were significantly lower.

Initially, Sweden's state epidemiologist, Anders Tegnell, admitted that the controversial decision not to impose strict public health measures had led to too many deaths, without any notable gains.[16] But Tegnell would later double down and defend his country's approach, suggesting that if or when there was a second wave, Sweden would have a high level of herd immunity and therefore a low number of cases compared to nearby countries like Finland, where a lockdown was strictly enforced.

But Tegnell's hopes that Sweden's anti-lockdown approach during the first wave would avert a second were dashed in the fall, when new infections and hospital admissions surged. By early November, the rate of hospitalizations and new infections was climbing faster than in any other European country. If Sweden's second wave was expected to feature relatively fewer cases because of an assumed higher level of community immunity, the strategy had failed. The country's death rate per capita was more than ten times that of neighbouring Norway, where strict public health measures had been imposed during the first wave, and approximately five times that of its other Nordic neighbours, like Denmark.[17] The COVID-19 second wave hit Sweden much harder than authorities had expected, and herd immunity had not been achieved.

In the United States, the lack of a nationwide strategy and the politicization of COVID response led to vastly different approaches to lockdown and other public health measures in different states. Largely divided by political ideology, jurisdictions led by Democrats generally complied with public health measures, whereas those led by Republicans defied them. Even as Florida hit record daily coronavirus death tolls, one sheriff ordered his officers not to wear face masks and banned them from his office. By September, as the world death rate approached one million, over 200,000 had been recorded in the US—the highest death rate per capita in the world.

This chaotic and haphazard response to dealing with the coronavirus led to the suggestion that the US could be viewed as an unplanned experiment in herd immunity. Eight months into the pandemic, White House officials even suggested that this was a strategy they were contemplating—a statement that provoked strong condemnation from many prominent doctors and scientists.[18] Reaching herd immunity by removing social distancing and other public health measures and unleashing the virus on the US population "would lead to the deaths of hundreds of thousands of Americans," William Hanage, an associate professor of epidemiology at Harvard University, commented.

One argument against allowing COVID-19 to run rampant

in communities is that the more times a virus replicates, the more opportunities there are for mutations to occur. We know that RNA viruses frequently mutate, and COVID-19 is an RNA virus. But as we have seen, it has some capacity to repair mutations and is therefore unlikely to be as unstable as flu viruses are, for example. But mutations in the original virus that was discovered in Wuhan in 2019 have consistently been observed.[19]

Most mutations do not cause a virus to become more virulent. In fact, they may weaken it. However, the likelihood of a mutation that makes COVID-19 more dangerous or infectious obviously gets greater the more the virus is passed from one person to another.

CONVALESCENT SERUM AND NEUTRALIZING ANTIBODIES

The plasma of patients who have recovered from infection—convalescent serum—contains neutralizing antibodies that can be harvested and given to someone who is still battling the infection. These antibodies protect just like infection or vaccine-induced antibodies, with the added advantage that they are available to fight infection immediately—there is no waiting period as there would be following either infection or vaccination. This is called "passive immunization."

Passive immunity is essential for the health and development of infants. A mother "passes" immunity against a wide variety of microbial pathogens to the fetus developing in her womb. Breast-feeding continues the passage of ready-made antibodies from the mother to the child, protecting the infant while its immune system is immature and it is most vulnerable to infection.

In the treatment of infection, passive immunization has a long history of use. Until the development of vaccines and antimicrobials, it was used with some success to treat a wide range of infections, including scarlet fever, mumps, measles, chickenpox and meningitis.[20] During the Spanish flu pandemic (1918–19), patients treated with convalescent serum showed significantly reduced mortality if the serum was given promptly.[21] Today, convalescent serum is still used to treat people after they have been exposed to untreatable infections like rabies.

Many patients who have recovered from COVID-19 have eagerly donated blood in the hope that the antibodies they produced to fight the virus could be harvested and used to help someone else. Convalescent serum containing neutralizing antibodies from recuperated COVID-19 patients appears safe, but it has not been shown to be consistently effective in decreasing the viral load and reducing mortality.[22]

The technology exists to make laboratory versions of naturally occurring antibodies against COVID-19. Called "monoclonal antibodies," they bind to viruses and prevent them from attaching and entering cells and initiating the cycle of infection just as effectively as natural antibodies from an infected or vaccinated person would do. In 1984, the Nobel Prize in Physiology or Medicine was awarded jointly to three immunologists—Niels Jerne, Georges Köhler and César Milstein—the latter two for developing monoclonal antibodies.

Monoclonal antibodies are made by immunizing a mouse with an antigen—in the case of COVID-19, with the virus itself or part of the virus. The mouse will then produce B cells that can be collected and grown in the laboratory to produce neutralizing antibodies against the virus. Normally, such cells are short-lived, and the amount of antibody they produce is therefore limited. Köhler and Milstein had the brilliant idea of fusing the antibody-producing B cells to a mouse cancer cell from a cancer called myeloma. These hybrid cells produce the required antibodies, but have the added advantage that they are immortal, so antibodies can be harvested in bulk.

Multiple clinical trials are underway to test the efficacy and safety of these laboratory-manufactured antibodies. If successful, they could be welcome additions to a growing armamentarium of first-line treatments.[23] When, in October, US president Donald Trump became ill with COVID-19, he received an experimental monoclonal antibody cocktail as part of his treatment. Pharmaceutical companies producing these antibodies have filed for emergency use while the results of clinical trials are still underway. Only time will tell how effective they are, or if they have any serious side effects.

MEDICATIONS AND COVID-19

COVID-19 is a novel virus, and to date no ready-made drug has been shown to prevent or treat it. Some existing antivirals have, however, been shown to be minimally effective, and they are being tested in clinical trials. Antivirals are best used early in infection when the viral load is low—that is, when the virus has not yet had a chance to infect too many cells and make too many copies of itself.

In severely ill patients, we have seen that the immune system itself becomes overactive and a cytokine storm develops. At this point, treatments are likely to be more beneficial if they are aimed at controlling the immune response itself, rather than the virus. Steroids are drugs that are frequently used in autoimmune diseases like rheumatoid arthritis or ulcerative colitis for their anti-inflammatory and immunosuppressant activities. They are also used to treat severely ill patients with sepsis, but with varying results.[24]

In a clinical trial in the UK, dexamethasone—a cheap and readily available steroid—was shown to reduce mortality by about one-third in COVID-19 patients on ventilators, and by about one-fifth in patients requiring only oxygen.[25] But the treatment had little effect on those not needing oxygen or ventilator support, a predictable outcome given that individuals with less severe disease presumably have not progressed to the stage where their immune systems are overreactive.

One trick that helps the novel coronavirus inflict so much damage is its ability to inhibit interferon production.[26] If administered before or soon after infection, interferons could tame the virus before it causes serious disease. Interferons have been used for decades for their immune-enhancing properties against infectious diseases like hepatitis, certain cancers, and autoimmune diseases like multiple sclerosis, and their safety is well established.

In the early stages of the pandemic, a hospital in China's Hubei province gave daily interferon nose drops to 2,415 front-line medical workers. Despite being in close contact with the virus, none of these workers apparently became infected.[27] An ongoing trial of inhaler steroids in the UK has shown that COVID-19 patients given inhaled interferon appear less likely to develop severe disease and to recover faster. The drug appears to restore the lung's immune response. Those given the treatment early reduced their odds of being hospitalized or developing severe disease compared with those given a placebo.[28] Many other clinical trials are underway to evaluate the effectiveness of interferons in COVID-19 infection.

However, with all of the many drugs currently being tested, researchers have cautioned that timing may be important. Andreas Wack, an immunologist at the Francis Crick Institute in the UK, quoted in the magazine *Science*, said, "Every study in every species has shown that if you induce interferons before [a] virus comes in, the virus loses. The earlier you can give it [interferon], the better, and the best thing you can do is to give it before the virus is there."[29] Several recent animal studies suggest that interferon given late in the disease, when the immune system is already in overdrive, could cause more harm than good.[30]

It is also conceivable that giving steroids too early could be a mistake, supressing immune responses before they get a chance to do their job. C-reactive protein (CRP) is a laboratory measure of inflammation. It climbs when inflammatory cytokines, especially interleukin-6, are increasing. One study found that when patients came to hospital with CRP levels of 20 mg/dL or more, they benefited from steroid treatment. But if CRP was less than 10 mg/dL, giving steroids was harmful, increasing the risk of mechanical ventilation and mortality.[31]

In the fall of 2020, as a second wave of COVID-19 hit Canada and other countries, one hopeful sign emerged: doctors were gaining a better handle on how best to treat patients. As cases once more skyrocketed, mortality rates in many areas appeared relatively well contained. While no single drug appeared to be a game changer, doctors were learning which drugs might help, and in which patients they might prevent the relentless march of COVID-19 from mild to severe or fatal disease.

VACCINE DEVELOPMENT AND COVID-19

While convalescent serum, monoclonal antibodies and the repurposing of existing drugs, used alone or in combinations, may all prove some help in treating this novel coronavirus, it is likely that community spread will only be halted—and the pandemic ended—once a vaccine becomes available.

It often takes many years of development and testing to show that a vaccine is both safe and effective. In fact, 90 per cent of all vaccines that start clinical trials never come to market at all, either because they failed to elicit a reliable immune response or because they were found to be unsafe.[32] The first effective mumps vaccine was developed in record time, and it still took four years. With a pandemic on our hands, the need for a successful vaccine was urgent—we could not wait a decade or two, or even four years.

One way to speed things up is to have a number of different scientific groups working on as many different approaches to developing a vaccine as possible. At the start of the pandemic, more than 150 groups began working to develop a coronavirus vaccine, with the WHO coordinating global efforts.

There are many different methods that can be used to produce a vaccine. One approach is to use the whole organism, but kill it with heat or chemicals, and use that as the inoculum. Or a virus can be weakened (attenuated) by growing it in the laboratory for many generations until a mutation occurs that makes the virus less likely to cause disease.

Another approach takes genes from a virus and inserts them into a weakened unrelated virus like the measles or a flu virus—called the vector—to get the pathogen genes into a host cell. Once they are inside a cell, the genes will produce coronavirus proteins, and these in turn will stimulate the immune system to make anti-coronavirus antibodies. Such vaccines are called "viral-vector vaccines." Other vaccines use fragments of coronavirus proteins, generally the spike protein, and inject them directly to elicit an immune response. In some cases, the empty shell of the coronavirus, which is not infective as it contains no genetic material, may be used.

One of the earliest vaccine research teams out of the gate, at Oxford University in the UK, began working on a vaccine early in January 2020. Partnering with AstraZeneca, a British-Swedish drug company, their vaccine used a viral-vector approach, with a chimpanzee adenovirus as the vector. In July, the first paper on the use of the vaccine was published. One thousand volunteers received a single dose of the vaccine. Participants were then followed for twenty-eight days and monitored for side effects and immune responses.[33]

No serious adverse events were noted—the most common were fatigue, headache and local tenderness at the site of vaccination, but these were tolerable. The vaccine stimulated a strong immune response, and volunteers who received the vaccine generated both antibodies and an "excellent" T cell response. The level of antibodies seen in the trial was similar to those seen in convalescent serum after natural infection.

A different approach to vaccine development involves injecting a synthetic version of part of the virus's genetic material—messenger RNA (mRNA)—that instructs the host cell to make infectious proteins. The host cells then follow the mRNA's instructions to create some of the virus's proteins, which the immune system detects; it then starts to produce a defensive antibody response. These mRNA vaccines are quick to produce, but the technology they use is new and, up to this point, no mRNA vaccine has ever been approved for use in humans.

By November 2020, two drug companies—Pfizer and its German partner BioNTech, and Moderna—announced they had developed mRNA vaccines against the virus that causes COVID-19. In early clinical trials, both vaccines, which were given in two doses, showed similar and excellent protection rates of 95 per cent. Close on their heels, more data on the more traditionally manufactured Oxford–AstraZeneca vaccine was published, showing that it provided 70 per cent protection. Researchers believed the protection rate could be improved by tweaking the vaccine dose: some of their volunteers who had been mistakenly given a half-sized first dose, followed by a full-sized second dose, achieved 90 per cent effectiveness.

WHO GETS THE VACCINE FIRST?

These early results were seen as a triumph. After all, we were only ten months into the pandemic. Scientific partnerships, as well as huge financial investments by governments, had produced results in record time. But it was one thing to develop vaccines; quite another entirely to get large portions of the global population actually vaccinated. Many logistical challenges had yet to be overcome before vaccination could begin on a mass scale.

The vaccine needed to be manufactured in bulk and then distributed. Distribution of the two mRNA vaccines would be problematic. One of them, by Pfizer, needed to be transported and stored at minus 70 degrees Celsius; the other, by Moderna, at minus 20. The Oxford–AstraZeneca vaccine was a little less of a challenge, since it could be stored in a regular refrigerator. It was also cheaper and easier to get to every corner of the world than the two mRNA vaccines.

By the end of October, Health Canada regulators were reviewing clinical trial data for all three of these new vaccines, the government having already signed agreements to buy promising vaccine candidates. In fact, Canada was better placed than most other developed countries, having pre-ordered sufficient supplies to eventually vaccinate 100 per cent of the population several times over. Public health officials had stocked up on needles and syringes to prepare for the first rollout.

But at first, limited supplies would be available and would have to be prioritized. The vaccine would therefore be targeted to those most likely to get the virus, such as health-care workers. Also at the front of the line were those at high risk of transmitting the disease, such as workers in long-term care homes, police, firefighters and other essential workers, as well as those most vulnerable to severe disease—the elderly and anyone with compromised immune systems.

There were also assurances that those with limited access to health care, such as Indigenous populations, would be a top priority for the Canadian government. What was difficult to estimate was how long it would be until mass vaccination had taken place and Canada had achieved the herd immunity threshold (between 60 and 70 per cent) the WHO has estimated would be needed to vanquish the virus.

In the meantime, the public health measures that were already in place—physical distancing, mask wearing, regular handwashing and avoiding crowds—would have to remain in place and be stringently observed until mass vaccination had taken place. Help might be coming soon, but it wasn't here yet.

LESSONS FROM HISTORY: THE CRIPPLING VIRUS

In 1910, a young girl living in Hamilton, Ontario, became sick with an illness initially thought to be rabies—a deadly viral disease that affects the nervous system and is almost universally fatal. But after she died, it was discovered that she did not have rabies, but another viral disease that affects the nervous system: polio. Although cases of polio have been recorded from antiquity, and outbreaks had been happening in Europe since the 1800s, this is thought to be the first recorded case of polio in Canada. Successive waves of infection followed, with the most severe outbreaks occurring between the 1930s and late 1950s.

Mainly affecting children under the age of five, polio is highly contagious. However, in past outbreaks, the majority of patients—around 95 per cent—were asymptomatic, although they were shedding the virus and were capable of passing it on to others.[34] Around 4 to 8 per cent of those with clinical signs of infection had minor symptoms—mainly mild gastroenteritis or respiratory symptoms—and recovered in about a week. However, a small proportion went on to get more serious disease, where the virus invaded the nervous system, damaging nerve cells called "motor neurons." Motor neurons activate muscles, and when they are damaged, muscles are paralyzed. In one in two hundred of those who got severe paralytic disease, the damage was permanent.[35]

During the 1950s, children who had recovered from a severe case of polio could often be identified by the metal leg braces they had to wear because their leg muscles had wasted and were too weak to support them. Muscles of the heart and the chest wall muscles—the intercostal muscles—could also be affected. Since intercostal muscles help expand and contract the lungs to facilitate breathing, damage to these muscles left some patients unable to breathe by themselves. They survived only by spending weeks or months in an "iron lung"—a metal chamber that encased the entire body except for the head. These fearsome capsules worked the lungs mechanically until, hopefully, the patient recovered sufficiently to be able to breathe unaided.

When vaccines against the polio virus became available in the 1950s, the incidence of polio in Canada fell rapidly, with the last case reported in 1977. In 1994, the WHO certified that Canada was free of polio, and since then only occasional sporadic cases have been seen, in Canadians returning from countries where polio is still prevalent. Polio cannot be cured, but it can be prevented through vaccination.

Unfortunately, for some of those who seemed restored to full health after a battle with polio, the story was not over. Decades later, they began to suffer from progressive weakness and pain in muscles and joints in what became known as post-polio syndrome. In post-polio syndrome, there can be renewed muscle wasting, and most sufferers report extreme fatigue and exhaustion with the slightest physical exertion. Post-polio syndrome is most likely to occur in those who originally suffered from the most severe disease—and, ironically, in those who made the best recovery.

What causes these symptoms many years after the original infection? Since weakness and wasting of muscles are both prominent features of the syndrome and of the disease itself, it might seem reasonable to assume that the polio virus had reactivated. However, post-polio syndrome is not contagious, and a more likely explanation is that the problem lies with damage originally inflicted by the polio virus on nerve cells.

Nerve cells, also called "neurons," are the main cells of the neurological system and are responsible for carrying information throughout the body. A single neuron does nothing by itself—it needs to communicate with other neurons, passing messages from one cell to another through branches called "dendrites" that radiate out from the body of the neuron, spreading out much like the branches or roots of a tree. The polio virus causes extensive damage to these dendrites, and this interferes with motor neuron function.

To compensate, remaining neurons sprout copious new dendrites, and the neurons enlarge, enabling muscles to recover and work again. But now the nerve cell has expanded considerably and requires a lot more nutrition to maintain these extra dendrites. If this nutrition is not supplied, it can lead to the gradual deterioration of the new dendrites and, eventually, to the death of the neuron itself.[36]

Although it's not life-threatening, post-polio syndrome is very debilitating. Symptoms can significantly interfere with quality of life, and patients require ongoing medical treatment and support. Muscle weakness can affect many bodily functions: weakness in respiratory muscles compromises lung function, affecting sleep and daytime energy; difficulty swallowing can cause choking and aspiration of food into the lungs, leading to pneumonia.[37]

Post-polio syndrome can occur in anyone who survived polio, even those who originally experienced only mild disease.

COVID-19 AND THE "LONG-HAULERS"

Once a patient with COVID-19 was out of danger and had tested negative for the virus, it was assumed they had recovered. But the actual lived experience of many of these "recovered" patients tells a different story. Many had experienced blood clots that caused strokes and heart attacks, lung scarring or kidney failure during their illness. Experts expected that these patients could be left with lifelong health problems from damage to major organs, including but not restricted to their lungs. These consequences of infection were not just seen in older patients, but in some younger ones too.

But as more and more cases of COVID-19 infection were documented, it became clear that while some patients recovered reasonably quickly, in others mysterious symptoms were lingering months after they were considered COVID-free. Symptoms ranged from crippling exhaustion, brain fog, persistent muscle weakness and difficulty breathing to intermittent fevers and chills.

Post-viral syndromes are not unknown in medicine, and it is entirely possible that something similar to what happened after polio could be happening after COVID-19. The closely related SARS virus that appeared on the scene in 2002 left some people with persistent fatigue, muscle pain, depression and disrupted sleep, and unable to work as long as thirteen to thirty-six months after infection, according to one Toronto study.[38] However, only about eight thousand people were diagnosed with SARS worldwide, so the unfortunate ones who developed lingering symptoms were happily few.

However, as the COVID-19 numbers spiked alarmingly in the autumn of 2020 and the numbers of infected individuals surged worldwide, the number of "long-haulers" may be expected to increase, too, potentially leaving a trail of medical, social and economic distress behind, long after the pandemic comes under control.

PART II

THE WELL-FED IMMUNE SYSTEM

CHAPTER FOUR

Medicine and the Lost Art of Nutrition

Nutrition is a cornerstone that affects and defines the health of all people, rich and poor. It paves the way for us to grow, develop, work, play, resist infection and aspire to the realization of our fullest potential as individuals and societies. —*World Health Organization, Nutrition, Health and Human Rights (2003 report)*

During the first wave of the pandemic, it became clear that although the severity of COVID-19 was greatest in the elderly, another group was also at high risk: those with pre-existing chronic diseases. Chronic diseases are conditions that are long-lasting and persistent and require ongoing medical attention. They don't spontaneously disappear.

Unlike infectious diseases, chronic diseases cannot be transmitted from one person to another. Nor can vaccines be developed to prevent them. In Canada, an estimated one in three people lives with at least one chronic disease.[1] Conditions that appeared to increase the risk and severity of COVID-19 included type 2 diabetes, obesity, high blood pressure and other heart conditions, chronic obstructive pulmonary disease (COPD), chronic kidney disease and cancer.

All of these conditions have been shown to be associated with inadequate diets and malnutrition, either as a cause or consequence of the disease.[2] We normally associate the word "malnutrition" with undernutrition or starvation. However, malnutrition also applies to overconsumption of calories, protein or fat and frequently results in overweight or obesity.

A well-primed immune response depends on good nutrition to function, and malnutrition is known to increase susceptibility to infections. In turn, infection can aggravate malnutrition, since it increases the body's demand for nutrients. This creates a vicious cycle, further increasing vulnerability to infection.[3]

In Canada, malnutrition is much more widespread than we would like to believe. A cross-Canada study conducted in eighteen hospitals screened patients for malnutrition on admission and found 45 per cent of them to be malnourished. Those who were malnourished had significantly longer hospital stays than those who were not.[4]

Malnutrition is very common in the elderly, too, especially those in residential care.[5] At one long-term care hospital in Toronto, undernutrition was reported in 45 per cent of residents, and in 18 per cent, the malnutrition was severe.[6] And it's not just because older people have less interest in food. A recent European study found the prevalence of undernutrition in the elderly to be 28 per cent in hospitals, 17.5 per cent in residential care and 8.5 per cent for those living in the community.[7] Similar data can be found for the UK, Australia and other developed countries.[8]

The immune system is an exquisitely sensitive indicator of the adequacy of nutritional intake. Decades ago, immunologists established that immune responses depend on ample intakes of protein, essential fats and specific vitamins and minerals.[9] During the pandemic, an unprecedented number of new scientific publications were rushed into print or appeared online. A search of the medical literature at the end of November 2020 revealed that out of more than eighty-three thousand new studies published on COVID-19, less than 2 per cent were concerned about nutrition.

The few studies that were done found that malnutrition was common in COVID patients admitted to intensive care units, and was associated with significantly poorer outcomes.[10] But in general, the importance of developing nutritional strategies to support immune function amid the pandemic, and possibly prevent the onset of severe infection, received very little attention.

A TALE OF TWO DIETS

The man waiting for me in my office was familiar. I had seen him when he accompanied his wife, a recovering cancer patient, to her dietary appointments. Now John was here on his own behalf, wondering if diet could help him get his elevated cholesterol under control. Recently retired from a physically demanding job, John was now living a more sedentary life, and in six months he had packed about ten kilograms onto his previously lean frame.

He and his wife were generally health-conscious and appeared to eat well—plenty of fresh vegetables, good-quality proteins and healthy fats—and he had started to go to the gym regularly. But his cholesterol continued its stubborn climb. Before putting him on cholesterol-reducing drugs, John's doctor had agreed to let him try changing his diet. If, after six months, diet had not helped, John accepted that he would need medication. As they parted, the doctor wished his patient good luck, but added, "I don't think this will work. I have rarely seen high cholesterol come down with diet alone."

Leafing through the diet sheets he had been given, John's heart sank. Many of the foods he would have to restrict were regular items on the family menu, and cutting them out would be a sacrifice. He would have to avoid foods high in cholesterol, especially eggs. He and his wife kept a few chickens in the garden, and he enjoyed a fresh egg every morning for breakfast. He would also have to cut out all traces of fat, particularly saturated fats like butter. Dairy products like milk and yogurt were OK, provided they were fat-free.

Wondering if there was another dietary approach or some dietary supplement that might help, his wife encouraged him to consult with me.

I had to agree with the doctor: the diet John had been given was not going to do the trick. The fat-as-a-cause-of-heart-disease hypothesis that had persisted for half a century was no longer supported by evidence.[11] And eggs were not the unhealthy foods we'd been led to believe: over the years, many research studies had shown that cutting out cholesterol-rich eggs had little impact on blood cholesterol.[12] I suggested that a sugar-free diet, low in starchy carbohydrates like bread and pasta, with lots of vegetables, sufficient protein and good fats at each meal would be more likely to help. John admitted to having a sweet tooth, and since his retirement he had eaten more bread and cookies than before and often had a handful of candies in his pocket.

Cutting back on these foods would increase his HDL (the so-called "good cholesterol"), I told John, and lower his triglycerides.[13] Triglycerides are measured along with cholesterol, and high blood levels increase the risk of heart disease. Any excess calories we eat are converted into triglycerides, which are then stored in fat cells as future sources of energy. Excess calories from fat, yes, but also from the foods many people overindulge in—the bread and cookies John loved.

I told John he could continue his daily egg, and have butter on his vegetables. As for zero-fat dairy, the research showed quite the opposite of what the diet sheets suggested: compared with full-fat milk and yogurt, skim milk and zero-fat yogurt actually *increased* rather than decreased cholesterol.[14] I also suggested that he take some vitamin supplements, including vitamin D, since low blood levels of D were known to be linked to higher cholesterol.[15]

I explained to him that cholesterol is found in many foods, especially egg yolks. But the cholesterol in his laboratory tests had mainly been produced by his own liver. Convincing studies had shown that in healthy people, reducing dietary cholesterol had no impact at all on blood levels.[16] And an increasing number of studies suggested that diets low in carbohydrate, rather than fat, were a more effective route to go when trying to get cholesterol production back under control.[17]

Six months later, John was back in the doctor's office, and his cholesterol was checked again. All measures were now normal. He was also back to his previous weight. As he left the office this time, John's doctor shook his hand. "Congratulations," he said. "I don't know how you did it, but you did it and I'm delighted!"

Back at my office, John wanted to know why the dietary advice I had given him, which had worked well, was so different from the diet sheets he had received. With only a few moments left before the end of our appointment, all I could say was, "It's complicated."

FOOD AS MEDICINE

Hippocrates (460–370 BC), the Greek physician and father of scientific medicine, said, "Let food be thy medicine and medicine be thy food." More than two thousand years later, modern medicine is finally recognizing that what we eat plays a major role in the development of chronic disease. Obesity, heart disease, diabetes, cancer, osteoporosis, chronic lung disease, kidney disease and dementia are all now considered diet-related diseases, and suboptimal nutrition is emerging as a leading cause of poor health.[18]

So, if food is medicine, why is there so little emphasis on it in doctors' offices? Many patients are eager to discover strategies they could use to improve their health, and consider their doctor the obvious source of trustworthy information.[19] But often, the only nutritional advice they receive is out of date and unlikely to be helpful.

At the heart of the problem lies the fact that little attention is paid to nutrition during a doctor's medical training. In 1985, the National Academy of Sciences in the United States recommended that a minimum of twenty-five hours should be allocated to nutrition in the curriculum. Twenty years later, only 27 per cent of American medical schools met even these meagre requirements, and the average was just 19.6 hours.[20] As a result, most doctors are not equipped with the knowledge or skills they need to effectively communicate dietary advice to their patients.

In Canada, the vast majority of medical students say they have insufficient up-to-date nutritional knowledge to properly counsel patients and that more time needs to be allocated to nutrition during their training.[21] The situation is not unique to North America, but is also a common complaint from medical students in other developed countries like the UK, Australia[22] and Japan.[23]

Historically, medical education has been biased towards identifying diseases and therapeutic interventions to control disease
processes rather than preventing disease itself through diet and
lifestyle interventions. The natural first choice to treat undesirable cholesterol levels in patients is therefore to prescribe one of
several drugs that will effectively suppress cholesterol production. Without training and competency in the field of nutrition,
it's not surprising that dietary interventions based on up-to-date
evidence—interventions that could also be effective—are so
rarely considered.[24]

WHEN WE TALK ABOUT NUTRITION, WHAT DO WE MEAN?

In talking about the impact of food on health, two words—"diet"
and "nutrition"—are often used interchangeably. But they do not
mean the same thing. According to the dictionaries, the word
"diet" simply describes the types of foods that people regularly
eat; or it may refer to an eating plan adopted to lose weight or to
address a specific medical problem—a low sodium diet for high
blood pressure, for example.

Unlike "diet," the word "nutrition" describes something altogether different. It is not just a catalogue of foods commonly
eaten; it also refers to whether or not those foods actually benefit our health. Although there are many dictionary definitions,
I find it difficult to imagine a better or more comprehensive one

than that of Sir Robert McCarrison, a British army doctor and nutritionist working in India in the early part of the twentieth century. Addressing a meeting of the British Medical Association in 1936, he asked his audience:

And what is "nutrition"? It is not merely "food," nor "that which nourishes," as some lay dictionaries define it. It consists in the taking in and assimilation through chemical changes—metabolism—of materials with which the tissues of the body are built, their waste removed, and their deterioration prevented; by which the processes of the body are regulated and coordinated, and from which energy is liberated for the internal and external work of the body.

And that's it in a nutshell. Each and every day, food must provide the raw materials needed not only for the structural upkeep of our bodies, but also for the regulation of countless body processes, such as blood pressure, cholesterol or blood sugar levels. Only from food can we obtain sufficient protein to repair and maintain organs and tissues. Only from food can we obtain critical fats that keep our brains working efficiently. Only from food do most of us get enough of the vitamins and minerals needed to control such vital processes as the rhythmic beating of the heart or the effective use of calories for energy.

As summed up by McCarrison, faulty nutrition leads to faulty functioning (such as cardiac arrhythmias), faulty structures (for example, osteoporotic bones), faulty health (the inability to fight viruses and win) and, ultimately, disease. Placing nutrition at the very heart of medicine, McCarrison argued, would result in the most rational approach to improving health, since there was no branch of medicine to which nutrition was not central.

McCarrison carried out extensive research on the then newly discovered vitamins and was one of the first to demonstrate links between poor nutrition and disease.[25] At that time, only severe nutritional-deficiency diseases like scurvy or rickets were considered matters of public health concern. But McCarrison's work showed that "minor manifestations of ill health"—troublesome but not life-threatening symptoms like fatigue, susceptibility to infection, impaired fertility, slow growth in children and poor wound healing—were also signs of deficiencies, and often harbingers of serious problems yet to come.[26] They were the red flags signalling that diet was inadequate and failing to provide optimal amounts of essential nutrients, and we ignored them at our peril.

McCarrison was the recipient of many prestigious scientific awards, and his work was widely published in medical journals. However, the clinical relevance of his work went unrecognized by the medical profession and there was no attempt to put into practice the lessons learned from the research of his day. His voice was ignored by medical schools, as were the voices of other eminent nutrition researchers of the time, and little of the new research was integrated into the medical curriculum. And so, the opportunity was missed to place nutrition where it should be: at the very heart of medicine.

Since then, medical schools have recognized that they need to pay more attention to nutrition education, but with competing demands for professional development time due to ever-changing guidelines on patient care, drug prescribing practices and new technologies, space is limited in the curriculum for a thorough grounding in nutrition.

Now we are in a crisis situation, where doctors and doctors-in-training lack the time or skills they need to be able to offer reliable preventative nutritional care to their patients. And all this in an age where most of the diseases doctors are expected to treat are known to be diet-related.[27]

WE ARE WHAT WE EAT

The average adult human body contains an estimated ten trillion cells, divided into some two hundred different types. Apart from some cells of nervous tissue and skeletal muscle, which generally do not increase in number after birth, new cells are continuously being formed.

Without this process of cell renewal, cells that are damaged or worn out would not be replaced. As a consequence, the tissues and organs they were part of would be weakened and ultimately become diseased. Even when we are healthy, the daily requirement to make new cells is estimated to be the equivalent of replacing the weight of an average adult body in new cells every eighteen to twenty-four months.[28]

In tissues that bear the daily brunt of wear and tear, cells need to be replaced at a fairly fast rate. Skin cells, for example, are subjected to constant friction. Flakes of dry skin are simply dead skin cells, and these have to be promptly replaced to preserve skin health. The average replacement time for a skin cell is three days. Other cells have varying lifespans. Red blood cells, for instance, last about three to four months. But cells that line the gastrointestinal tract are subjected to trauma each and every time we eat, and it has been estimated that there is almost complete replacement of the cellular lining of the entire gastrointestinal tract every two to six days.[29]

First-responder immune cells like neutrophils live only a few hours in the blood, and to replace them and keep innate immune responses well primed, the average adult must make approximately one hundred billion new neutrophils every day.[30] The timely replacement of healthy neutrophils therefore becomes a critical factor in mounting an immune response. Whatever their replacement rate, new cells cannot be manufactured without appropriate raw materials. Those raw materials are the protein and essential fats from diet, together with the vitamins and minerals needed to convert them into cells.

What happens when we do not consume enough of the raw materials to replace dead and dying cells, or when those raw materials are in an inferior form? Like a shipwrecked sailor stranded on a desert island who can make himself a shelter only with whatever materials he can find, the body can construct new cells only from the available food supply. Habitually making poor food choices will result in weak, poorly functioning cells, just as certainly as a lack of appropriate building materials means that the sailor can only build an insubstantial shelter that may offer him little protection in a storm.

An example of what can happen if the wrong cellular building materials are present in diet was seen when, during the 1960s, industrially created fats called "trans fats" began to increase dramatically in the food supply. Now banned in many countries, trans fats are molecularly altered fats that extend the shelf life of foods. Used in the manufacture of many commercial foods like margarine, crackers and cookies, they are still present in deep-fried foods, generated by the high cooking temperatures.

In cell membranes, trans fats can take the place of the essential omega-3 fats. This irreversibly changes the way cells communicate. Incorporated into the membranes of brain cells, for example, trans fats alter the ability of neurons to talk to one another, impacting mental performance.[31] When incorporated into the membrane of cells lining arteries—endothelial cells—trans fats promote cholesterol accumulation and increase the risk of heart disease.[32]

FORM AND FUNCTION

It's not just cell replacement that suffers when dietary intake of essential nutrients is inadequate. The connective tissue that provides the scaffolding and framework of the body also needs constant upkeep. Connective tissue comes in a wide variety of forms, performing a wide range of functions, but its main job is to support and connect organs and tissues. Structural connective tissue includes skin, bone and cartilage. The strength and resilience of cartilage in knees and hips, for example, depends on dietary protein and the availability of key vitamins and minerals for its repair and maintenance. Vitamins C, D and E, as well as the minerals copper, zinc and manganese, are all involved.[33]

For the brain to work, neurons need to be able to communicate with one another. They do this either in the form of electrical signals or by using chemical messengers called "neurotransmitters." Whether you are trying to learn something new, remember the name of an old friend or get a good night's sleep, all tasks executed by the brain rely on a continuous supply of several different neurotransmitters—dopamine for focus and concentration, serotonin for sleep, acetylcholine for memory. The manufacture and efficient release of these neurotransmitters depends on the availability of their precursor molecules—the food-derived building blocks from which they are made—in every meal. If the precursor to a neurotransmitter is not available, the brain cannot create that neurotransmitter.

For example, poor focus and concentration, combined with low mood or depression, are hallmarks of dopamine deficiency. To make sufficient dopamine to meet the brain's continuing needs, we need protein to provide dopamine's precursor, the amino acid tyrosine. A diet low in protein may not provide enough tyrosine to maintain high brain dopamine levels.[34]

We also need to take in enough of a variety of vitamins and minerals that are cofactors in the manufacture of dopamine. These include all the B vitamins—B_1, B_2, B_3, B_6, folic acid, B_{12} and the fatty B-like compound choline—vitamins C, D and E, and minerals that include calcium, magnesium, sodium, potassium, iron and zinc.[35] Insufficient blood levels of any one of these nutrients has been linked to depression.[36]

Hormones also act as messenger molecules. Manufactured in one part of the body, they travel to other parts, where they help control how cells and organs do their work. Thyroxine is a hormone made by cells in the thyroid gland—a small, butterfly-shaped gland that lies just under the skin, low down in the neck. Every cell in the body depends on thyroxine to regulate its metabolism, and without sufficient thyroxine, cell metabolism slows down, compromising a whole host of bodily functions.

The replacement of cells requires thyroxine, so signs of low thyroid function include hair loss and dry skin. Brain cells need thyroxine for neurotransmitter production, so other indications of sluggish thyroid activity include lethargy and depression. Thyroxine is also essential for reproduction and for the regulation of sex hormones, and low thyroid function can result in infertility and frequent miscarriages.[37]

Just as it is for dopamine, the building block for thyroxine is tyrosine, but the mineral iodine is also an essential component. Lack of either protein to provide tyrosine or of the essential trace mineral iodine will result in an underactive thyroid gland.[38]

Browsing through some files recently, I found an old newspaper clipping with the headline "Nation of gnashers shows stress of the 90s." The article goes on to describe the growing concern of dentists that serious damage to teeth is the price being paid for the increased workplace, financial and emotional stress of the 1990s.

Tooth grinding is also known as "bruxism." It usually happens during sleep, so it is beyond our conscious control. The force generated by bruxism can vary from three to ten times the force generated during normal chewing—enough to grind teeth over time into little more than stumps. Dentists usually prescribe night guards similar to the gum shields used by football players to be worn during sleep. This is not a cure, but it will help limit the damage done by intense grinding.

Regular grinding can also damage temporomandibular joints (TMJ)—small joints at the front of the ears where the lower jaw, or mandible, is attached to the skull. For chewing, swallowing and speaking to be comfortable, these joints need to be well cushioned by connective tissue, and regular grinding wears that tissue down. Tooth grinders often wake up in the morning with aching jaws and tight face muscles. Muscle relaxants before bed are usually prescribed for bruxism; if they don't work, injections of Botox—a toxin that partially paralyzes jaw muscles—may be offered. In some cases, antidepressant and anti-anxiety medicines may also be suggested.

Another debilitating problem that frequently coexists with

bruxism is restless legs syndrome (RLS)—an overwhelming and uncomfortable urge to move the legs that is only relieved by movement. It is generally accepted as a chronic condition. Low levels of the neurotransmitter dopamine are thought to be the root cause of RLS, so dopamine-enhancing drugs such as L-dopa, used in the treatment of Parkinson's disease,[39] or anti-anxiety medications like the benzodiazepines may be prescribed.[40] Both drugs have side effects: L-dopa can lead to worsening of symptoms, and long-term use of benzodiazepines should be avoided as they are addictive and are now known to increase the risk of dementia.[41]

A common and mostly overlooked cause of all three conditions—bruxism,[42] TMJ[43] and RLS[44]—is magnesium deficiency. Magnesium deficiency causes neuromuscular hyperexcitability—extreme overactivity of nerves, which in turn causes muscles to spontaneously contract and go into spasm.[45] By current estimates, at least 50 per cent of North Americans do not consume the daily recommended amounts of magnesium.[46]

Changes in farming practices over the years are partly to blame. The magnesium content of vegetables, a rich source of the mineral, has declined by 80 to 90 per cent over the last hundred years.[47] As far back as the 1930s, the alarm was being raised about the growing scarcity of magnesium and other minerals in food.

The alarming fact is that foods (fruits, vegetables and grains) now being raised on millions of acres of land that no longer contain enough of certain minerals are starving us—no matter how much of them we eat. No man of today can eat enough fruits and vegetables to supply his system with the minerals he requires for perfect health because his stomach isn't big enough to hold them.[48]

The processing of food further depletes already scarce magnesium, and ultra-processed foods that make up such a high proportion of modern diets in North America are seriously lacking in magnesium.[49] To add to the problem, the mineral is depleted by many widely used prescription medications.[50]

But a major factor impacting magnesium status is the significant and rapid loss of the mineral from the body due to stress.[51] All types of stress—workplace stress, exam stress, emotional stress, exposure to excessive noise, the stress of extreme physical activity or chronic pain, the stress of fighting infections—are known to be a serious drain on magnesium resources.[52]

The interaction of magnesium with stress works in two ways: while stress depletes magnesium, the deficiency itself increases anxiety and enhances uncontrolled hormonal response to stress. This creates a vicious feedback loop whereby stress depletes magnesium, but the ensuing magnesium deficiency further exacerbates stress.[53]

WHAT IS AN ESSENTIAL NUTRIENT?

So, is it a problem if medications are used to treat everyday conditions like restless legs or tooth grinding, instead of first trying to correct any likelihood of magnesium deficiency? Both will work, so does it matter which approach you take?

Magnesium is an essential nutrient. By definition, an essential nutrient is a substance we need for survival and optimal functioning, one that must be obtained from diet because we cannot synthesize it ourselves. Essential nutrients are therefore necessary for the continuity of life itself. This is not a matter for speculation or argument. The fact that most nations of the world stipulate a minimum daily intake of all the essential nutrients is an acknowledgement that if we regularly fall short in our consumption of any of them, there is a price to be paid.[54]

Magnesium deficiency is associated with high blood pressure, heart arrhythmias and heart attacks. A shortage of magnesium may also precipitate strokes.[55] Both blood sugar and insulin control require magnesium, and ensuring adequate intakes of the mineral may help head off the development of type 2 diabetes.[56] If bruxism or RLS indicates magnesium deficiency, then replenishing magnesium is likely not only to help with the immediate health problem, but also to have multiple benefits, preventing the onset or worsening of these other conditions. In the face of the diminishing content of magnesium in food, supplements are likely to be necessary.[57]

However, magnesium supplementation is tricky. Because of differences in genetic requirements,[58] the concurrent use of many magnesium-depleting drugs[59] and the continuous depletion of magnesium by stress,[60] each patient is likely to have different needs—sometimes dramatically different. Supplement recommendations therefore have to be tailored to the needs of each individual patient. There is no one-size-fits-all dose that will meet the needs of everyone.

Addressing an individual's unique nutritional needs is called "personalized nutrition"—currently a growing field in nutritional research.[61]

WHEN BLOOD TESTS DON'T HELP

Nutritional deficiencies are usually identified by clinically validated blood tests. When intake of vitamin C, vitamin D or iron is low, for example, it will be reflected in the amount of each nutrient present in blood, which can be tested, and any deficiency can be remedied. Unfortunately, blood tests are of little help in identifying shortfalls of magnesium.[62]

Only a tiny fraction of total body magnesium is present in blood—less than 1 per cent of total body stores. The remaining 99 per cent is found roughly divided between bone and different types of muscle. If blood levels drop, even momentarily, the body quickly shifts magnesium out of bone stores or muscle cells and into the blood. Blood levels therefore remain constant and rarely dip into the deficiency range, even in the presence of significantly inadequate dietary intake.[63]

There is a very good physiological explanation for why the body might want to maintain constant blood levels. Magnesium is indispensable to the relaxation of muscles after they contract.

The rhythmic beating of the heart depends on the smooth contraction and relaxation of cardiac muscle, and without sufficient magnesium, the heart would falter. So, the body will always prioritize scarce magnesium resources to maintain heart function.

Laboratory testing can be useful for detecting critically deficient magnesium stores; because low blood levels are so seldom seen in the general population, such a reading suggests either that body stores really have bottomed out, or that the normal physiological mechanism for shifting magnesium from body stores into the blood is compromised. Either way, low serum magnesium should be urgently corrected, since low levels are known to be linked to sudden cardiac arrest and heart attacks.[64]

Heart rhythm abnormalities like palpitations, arrhythmias and atrial fibrillation[65] are known to be linked to a shortage of magnesium. We notice this effect at work when we feel our heart "skipping a beat" if we are exposed to sudden magnesium-depleting stress. In chapter 6, we will explore alternative methods of identifying and correcting magnesium deficiency.

WHAT IS EVIDENCE-BASED NUTRITION?

From early in the twentieth century until the 1970s, a bland diet called the Sippy diet was used for the treatment of peptic ulcers. Named after the American internist Bertram Welton Sippy (1866–1924), the diet consisted of milk and cream every couple of hours for three days to keep stomach acid neutralized. After that, a few other bland foods like cereal, crackers and eggs were gradually introduced. Finally, small portions of puréed vegetables could be eaten.

Generations of gastroenterologists prescribed this diet, believing that it healed ulcers. It did relieve pain, but once fibre-optic technology became available and the inside of the stomach and small intestine could be directly visualized, it became clear that the diet was not healing ulcers. It was also clear that the diet could increase the risk of cardiovascular disease: patients on the Sippy diet were twice as likely to have heart attacks than ulcer patients who were not.[66]

This is just one example of a common medical protocol having to be discontinued when research proves that it is unreliable or even potentially harmful. To increase the effectiveness of clinical practice, a new discipline called "evidence-based practice" was introduced into medicine at the end of the twentieth century. Evidence-based practice requires that any medical procedure or drug have solid scientific data to prove it works. No assumptions; rather, hard evidence. In recent years, evidence-based practice has become the backbone of clinical medicine.

Randomized controlled trials (RCTs) are considered the gold standard in medical research. Originally introduced into clinical medicine when the antibiotic streptomycin was being tested for the treatment of tuberculosis in the 1940s, RCTs are studies that compare outcomes in patients or volunteers who have been randomly assigned to receive a drug or other intervention with those in patients or volunteers given a placebo—an inert substance unlikely to have any physiological effect. The advantage of an RCT is that it gives clear-cut answers: the only difference between the experimental and control group is that one gets the treatment and the other does not.

In recent years, the RCT has been borrowed from pharmaceutical research to study vitamins. However, vitamins are not drugs, and they do not work alone—rather, they depend on complex interactions with other nutrients for their function. Randomized controlled trials, while entirely appropriate for studying drugs, were never designed to study multiple interacting compounds. Indeed, it is impractical, if not impossible, to obtain reliable information on vitamins using this approach.

Proof of the fact that RCTs cannot be used to study complex interactions comes not from nutritional research, but from studying drugs. Many people take multiple drugs for different health conditions. This is called "polypharmacy." While each drug will have been tested separately, no one knows whether they are safe or efficacious when taken together—or indeed, if they might enhance each other when combined and improve clinical outcomes.

When researchers tried to see if they could design RCTs to test multiple drugs that could potentially be useful in combination, they showed just what an impossible task it would be. The researchers chose to study two conditions: Alzheimer's disease and ischemic stroke. At the time of the study, seven drugs had been approved for preventing or slowing progression in Alzheimer's disease, while five had been approved for treating ischemic stroke.

The researchers estimated that testing seven drugs in various combinations for Alzheimer's disease would require the enrollment of 63,500 patients in 127 individual clinical trials, and it would be 286 years before they would know which combination of the seven drugs, if any, showed the most benefit. Similarly, testing combinations of the five drugs used for ischemic stroke would necessitate thirty-one trials, enrolling 186,000 patients and lasting for 155 years.[67]

WE CAN'T STUDY NUTRIENTS ONE AT A TIME

Research into osteoporosis illustrates perfectly the folly of studying nutrients one at a time. Bones are highly dynamic structures, constantly being broken down and then rebuilt. The breakdown of bone plays an important role in normal metabolism, releasing magnesium and other minerals into the bloodstream when needed. Then, provided there is an adequate dietary provision of bone-building nutrients, the bones will be rebuilt. Osteoporosis arises when bone loss outpaces bone reconstruction.

All of the essential nutrients are needed for the maintenance of bone.[68] Protein, B vitamins and vitamin C are all needed to create the scaffolding to which the minerals attach to form a rigid structure. The main strengthening mineral in bone is calcium, and bones need plenty of this mineral. But calcium from diet or supplements will not be absorbed if there is a shortage of vitamin D, and vitamin D's activation in turn depends on the availability of magnesium. Sufficient vitamin K is then needed to attach calcium to bone. Other trace minerals like zinc, boron and manganese also have roles to play. So, for the building of strong bones in childhood and their upkeep throughout our lives, we are dependent on a continuing optimal intake of all essential nutrients. Not one, not two, but *all*.

Suppose an old boat had a number of holes in the bottom. Repairing one of those holes would not make the boat seaworthy; all holes would need to be fixed before the boat could be safely launched. Or imagine a leaky roof with several missing shingles. Replacing one shingle, or even a group of them, would not keep out the rain if all the missing shingles were not replaced.

And so it is with the essential nutrients. Without vitamin D, we cannot absorb calcium, the most abundant mineral in bone. In those who are vitamin D deficient, especially those living at more northerly latitudes, osteoporosis is a likely outcome. But taking vitamin D, or vitamin D with calcium, will not help much if we are short of any of these other critical bone-building nutrients.

So, when we talk about "evidence-based nutrition," we have to carefully scrutinize the methods used to arrive at such evidence. Nutritional research faces challenges that don't arise in drug trials, and methods designed to test drugs (RCTs) are poor tools when applied to studying vitamins. When we rely solely on RCTs as evidence, it is likely that the impact of nutrient shortfalls on our health is seriously underestimated.[69]

POOR NUTRITIONAL RESEARCH LEADS TO INCORRECT CONCLUSIONS

No one food contains all the essential nutrients in the amounts needed to sustain life, and no single vitamin, no matter how much of it we take, can compensate for deficiencies of other essential nutrients. But we persistently study single foods or isolated vitamins.

What happens when an RCT of a single nutrient proves to be of little or only marginal benefit? If the researchers failed to control for all other possible interacting nutrients—as we have seen, an impossible task—the study is meaningless, and the conclusions can and should be dismissed. Unfortunately, it is more likely the researchers will conclude that since their study showed no benefit, the nutrient in question is of no concern. This is not only an incorrect conclusion, but a dangerous one.

Dr. Michael Allan, a professor of family medicine at the University of Alberta, and his colleagues reviewed 1,600 studies on vitamin D, looking for evidence of benefits from vitamin D supplementation. They found some evidence that vitamin D used alone might help prevent falls and fractures in seniors, but the benefit was minimal. They found no evidence that vitamin D supplements could prevent cancer, heart disease or respiratory infections, or help in the treatment of rheumatoid arthritis, multiple sclerosis or depression.[70]

Commenting on the results to the media, Dr. Allan said, "Wouldn't it be great if there was a single thing that you or I could do to be healthy that was as simple as taking a vitamin every day? There is an appeal to it. There is a simplicity to it. But for the average person, they don't need it."[71] An unfortunate and simplistic conclusion.

Suppose you are a garage mechanic faced with a car that won't start. You suspect a faulty battery and replace it. But the car still won't start. Would you assume that the battery was unimportant and had no role to play in keeping the car on the road? Of course not, since you would know that there are many other reasons for engine failure: the ignition switch or starter motor might have failed, or maybe the fuel pump is faulty. Not until you had tested all the essential elements needed to keep the engine working would you know what was needed to get that particular car road-worthy again. And you would make sure that all the elements needed to keep the car running were optimized to prevent future problems.

And so it is with nutrition: deficiencies of any of the essential nutrients will cause vital metabolic processes to falter. But just as no single nutrient can shoulder all the blame for osteoporosis or depression, no single nutrient can be expected to correct complex health problems, including sluggish or inappropriate immune responses. To investigate the impact of vitamin D or any other single nutrient alone for immune health or disease prevention is a bit like employing a car mechanic who only bothers to check spark plugs—not the sort of mechanic who is going to help you keep your car in tip-top running order.

If we are to prioritize nutrition in disease treatment and

prevention, we must understand all of nutrition's working parts and their interactions, and find ways to optimize each of them.

NUTRIENTS MULTITASK; NUTRIENTS COOPERATE

While comparing the complexity of nutrient interactions in the human body to the complexity of a machine like a car is useful to illustrate the futility of single-nutrient research, it is an imperfect analogy, since it ignores one fact that adds another layer of complexity to the study of nutrition: all nutrients multitask. So, while each part of the car is designed to perform one (and only one) task, each essential nutrient has not one role to play in our physiology, but many.

In the early days of vitamin D research, its role in bone health was the only one considered. In recent years, this view has expanded, and it is now clear that vitamin D has a role to play in virtually every system of the body, including the immune system. The vitamin D receptor (VDR)—the docking molecule that binds the vitamin—is now known to be present on almost all cells, implying that vitamin D is involved in the functioning of those cells.

Most cells of the immune system express the VDR, including regulatory T cells, antigen-presenting cells, dendritic cells and macrophages.[72] Quoted in *Scientific American*, Carsten Geisler, a professor of international health, immunology and microbiology at the University of Copenhagen, put it this way:

When a T cell is exposed to a foreign pathogen, it has an immediate biochemical reaction and extends a signalling device or "antenna" known as a vitamin D receptor, with which it [searches] for vitamin D. This means that the T cell must have vitamin D, or activation of the cell will cease. If T cells cannot find enough vitamin D in the blood, they won't even begin to mobilize.[73]

If, in the absence of vitamin D, immune cells will not mobilize, it becomes imperative that we maintain good blood levels of vitamin D all the time, or else immune responses will definitely be compromised.

However, vitamin D alone is not enough for fully functional immunity; it also relies on the presence of various other micronutrients, including vitamins A, C, E, B_2, B_6 and B_{12}, folic acid, iron, selenium and zinc.[74] All the vitamin D in the world cannot compensate for deficiencies of any of these other nutrients.

The immune system is a very sensitive indicator of nutritional adequacy. A properly balanced diet, with an abundance of unprocessed foods like fruits and vegetables and whole grains, together with adequate intake of the essential nutrients—vitamin D, vitamin A, the B vitamins (folate, vitamin B_6 and vitamin B_{12}), vitamin C and the minerals iron, copper, selenium and zinc—all contribute to the normal functioning of the immune system.[75]

In the next chapters, we will look at ways to optimize diets and use nutritional supplements to fortify our immune system. Hopefully, we may be better prepared in future to deal with novel, potentially lethal pathogens.

CHAPTER FIVE

Good Food; Healing Food

I know of nothing so potent in maintaining good health in laboratory
animals as perfectly constituted food; I know of nothing so potent
in producing ill health as improperly constituted food. This, too, is
the experience of stockbreeders. Is man an exception to the rule so
universally applicable to the higher animals?
—*Sir Robert McCarrison (1878–1960)*

The summer of 2020 had been long and hot. Month by
month, the number of new COVID-19 cases decreased
substantially. In Toronto, everyone breathed a sigh of relief and
tried to make the most of the fine weather. Indoor dining was dis-
couraged, so makeshift patios popped up on sidewalks, in alleys
and in parking lots. The twinkling lights decorating these newly
carved-out restaurant spaces created an unusually festive atmosphere in the city. On weekends, some major roads were closed
to motor traffic, so that people could get outside and walk or bike
for exercise and still maintain physical distancing.

But many young people chose to ignore public health advice and congregated in large numbers at beach and house parties. Following some of these events, there were predictable spikes in infection rates, but since many of those testing positive were young adults who were less susceptible to serious disease, hospitalizations remained low. Then, as summer faded into autumn, the number of new cases began to increase—slowly at first, and then, by early November, dramatically. Worrisome rates of new infection were seen, not just in prior hot spots, but also in areas that had succeeded at keeping community spread low. The anticipated second wave was underway.

Now the disputes about how to manage this new surge began in earnest. Undoubtedly, the economy had suffered when nonessential businesses were shut down during the first wave, and we heard many heartbreaking stories about small businesses—restaurants, bars, fitness studios and clothing stores—having to shut their doors permanently.

Politicians in some jurisdictions took decisive action, implementing new lockdowns just as they had in the spring. In other regions, they dithered. We couldn't afford to revert to previous lockdowns, they argued. We would have to compromise, balancing the need to prevent infection against the needs of the economy. There were two fatal flaws with this argument: viruses don't compromise, and you can't run an economy with sick people. Tough measures would be needed if we were to face down the virus this time.

By the last week of November, Toronto was again back in

lockdown. This one, known as a circuit breaker, would be four weeks long—or two reproductive cycles of the virus, which had an incubation period of fourteen days. Non-essential businesses were closed; malls were shuttered. Shopping was limited to essential items only, and shopping for the holiday season, which had only just begun, faded from the main streets and shifted online.

At home, people could only mix with members of their own households. Visitors were forbidden. Church services, weddings and funerals were limited to a maximum of ten people, whether indoors or outdoors. There were stiff fines in place for breaking any of these regulations. This year, the holiday season was going to be very different.

AGING, CHRONIC DISEASE AND COVID-19

During the second wave, the elderly were still the most vulnerable. This shouldn't really have been a surprise, since the immune system is known to deteriorate with age. The older we get, the more susceptible we are to infection.

This gradual weakening of the immune system is called "immunosenescence," and it not only increases susceptibility to infection, it results in poorer responses to vaccination and increased prevalence of cancer and autoimmune diseases.[1] Immunosenescence is also known as "inflammaging" (inflammation + aging), since one of its hallmarks is chronic whole-body inflammation.[2] A surge in inflammation is part of the body's normal immune response.

The classical signs of inflammation—warmth, redness, swelling and pain—are all evidence that immune cells have mobilized and are gathering to deal with a pathogen, or to begin the repair of damaged tissues.

In healthy individuals, inflammation dies down after resolution of the infection or the injury that triggered it. But in inflammaging, the embers are not extinguished; a low-grade chronic inflammatory state smoulders on, causing ongoing tissue damage. Inflammaging accompanies all chronic diseases[3] and is also a major factor in the development and perpetuation of obesity.[4]

Most of the chronic conditions associated with persistent inflammation fall into the category of lifestyle diseases—conditions that can be blamed, at least in part, on habits and behaviours that are known to undermine health, such as poor diet, lack of exercise or smoking. For decades, we have been aware that smoking not only causes lung cancer, but is implicated in the development of all the main chronic diseases. It is sobering to learn that if we habitually make poor dietary choices, we increase the risk of future disease at least as much as if we smoked.[5]

"Most of our patients know that it's probably not a good idea to smoke, but I don't think they have a sense of the magnitude of the importance of the food choices they are making every day," said Michelle McMacken, assistant professor of medicine at the New York University School of Medicine. "Nearly half of all deaths due to heart disease, stroke and diabetes are due to poor, suboptimal diet."[6]

If poor nutrition is a major factor in the decline of immunity, could the right diet make a difference? Would improved nutrition dampen down inflammation and slow the progressive deterioration in immune health with age? The answer appears to be yes.[7] But the question is: which diet?

Do a Google search using the term "nutrition confusion" and you are likely to get in excess of thirty million hits, a number that clearly reflects the current uncertain state of play in the field of nutrition. The studies on diet and health are endless, but the advice that flows from them is often frustratingly contradictory. For every study that warns against the perils of coffee, there is another pointing to coffee as the key to cancer prevention and longevity. Eggs have been the victim of so many flip-flops on whether or not we should eat them, it's enough to make your head spin.

One reason may be the way in which much dietary research is carried out. Most large-scale dietary studies rely on self-reported food consumption. The quality of this research obviously depends on how accurately we can recall the types and amounts of food we have eaten. But how reliable is our food recall? When one group of women was asked to taste eight different fun snack foods (pretzels, M&M's, etc.) and then, one day later, recall the types and amounts of the foods they had eaten, most got it wrong. Either they couldn't recall all of the different items they'd consumed or they underestimated how much they had eaten.[8]

If it's so difficult to remember the sweet treats we ate yesterday, how likely is it that we can remember precisely how many eggs, how much dairy or any other food we have eaten over the past week, month, year or even longer? But that's exactly what studies based on food recall data expect us to do. Leaving aside difficulties with food recall, the main problem with studies of single foods is that we rarely consume foods one at a time, but as part of a mixed diet. So, no one can say whether it was the particular food under study, or other food items consumed at the same time as the study food, that was a problem. As we discussed in the last chapter, it's not just difficult to make sense of research that focuses on single components of diet, it's scientifically untenable.[9]

OBESITY—NOW AND THEN

Obesity has affected a small portion of populations for centuries, but rates were stable until the early 1980s, when a dramatic increase was seen in most industrialized countries, led by the United States. In underdeveloped countries, obesity was rare for much of the twentieth century. However, as these countries have adopted Western-style eating patterns, obesity is increasing there, too. In 2014, a major international study found that one-third of the world's population was overweight or obese, and 62 per cent of obese individuals lived in developing countries.[10] Obesity is now considered to be an even greater risk factor than smoking for developing chronic illnesses and for premature death.[11]

We define body weight as healthy or not using a measure called the body mass index (BMI), which relates weight to height and is an approximate measure of body fat. There are many online calculators to help you figure out your BMI. If it is between 18.5 and 24.9, your weight is considered normal; between 25.0 and 29.9, you are overweight; and a person with a BMI of 30.0 or higher is considered obese.

How weight is distributed also matters. Fat that is mainly on the hips and thighs—the so-called pear shaped body—is mainly subcutaneous. This type of fat prevents heat loss, acts as a barrier to infection and serves as a cushion against physical trauma. It is also a storage site for excess dietary calories. When present in normal amounts, subcutaneous fat is healthy. But excessive amounts increase the risk of all chronic diseases, especially type 2 diabetes and cardiovascular disease.

If you are apple-shaped, excess body fat is deposited around the waist and belly—so-called "visceral fat." Visceral fat is stored within the abdominal cavity, where it wraps around several vital organs, including the heart and liver. It can also build up in bone marrow and in arteries. Visceral fat is the most dangerous type of fat and is mainly responsible for inflammation and the adverse health effects of obesity. Lean, healthy individuals have very little visceral fat.

COVID, IMMUNITY AND THE
WEIGHT CONNECTION

Studies in both animals and in humans have shown that the more a person weighs, the more likely they are to succumb to infection— any infection. If you contract COVID, having a BMI between 30 and 40—or being extremely obese (a BMI of 40 or above)— increases your risk that the infection will be severe or fatal, according to the Centers for Disease Control and Prevention.

Once upon a time, excess body fat was thought of simply as stored excess calories. Not anymore. Along with a growing understanding of the hormonal and metabolic changes that accompany weight gain, scientists now have a better explanation for why visceral fat increases the risk of all chronic diseases and impacts immunity. Eating too much—more calories than we need for our metabolism to function—stimulates an immune response. In turn, an activated immune system generates inflammation.

Recent research has shown that immune cells, mainly macrophages, accumulate in visceral fat in both lean and obese individuals. However, in lean individuals, most of the macrophages play an anti-inflammatory role, whereas in obese individuals the macrophages are more likely to *promote* inflammation.[12] Excess visceral fat permanently pushes the immune system into a state of perpetual inflammation, releasing inflammatory cytokines into the bloodstream. In turn, excess cytokines cause tissue damage and impact the health of organs throughout the body.[13]

So, if your BMI is normal, are you protected from increased inflammation? Not necessarily. Even individuals of normal weight can have hidden excess visceral fat, which can be identified using CT or MRI scans. Examining individuals whose BMI was normal, but who had more than 30 per cent visceral fat, researchers found that they had increased blood levels of inflammatory cytokines, putting these "thin-on-the-outside, fat-on-the-inside" individuals at increased risk of diabetes, cardiovascular disease and cancer.[14]

As we have seen, the immune system is always active, quietly carrying out surveillance against cancer and infection. But during active infection, it goes into serious overdrive. This increased activity is accompanied by a dramatically increased demand for the nutrients the immune system depends on. And these nutrients can only come from the food we eat or, as we will see in the next chapter, dietary supplements.

A well-fed immune system is a well-functioning immune system, and the key to good defences against infection and inflammation depends not just on luck or good genes, but on whatever is in your lunch box or on your dinner plate.

COUNTERING INFLAMMATION: ANTIOXIDANTS TO THE RESCUE

At the root of inflammaging is the excessive production of molecules called "free radicals." Free radicals are short-lived, unstable molecules that are a product of normal cellular metabolism.

Most, but not all of the biologically significant free radicals are based on oxygen, and are called "reactive oxygen species" (ROS). At high concentrations, ROS and other free radicals are extremely toxic and can damage major components of cells—their RNA and DNA, and cell membranes. This damage, called "oxidative stress," plays a key role in the development of cancer and chronic health conditions.

Generally, viral infections ramp up the release of free radicals, and in the process, they deplete antioxidants. One possible explanation for the severity of COVID-19 in at-risk groups is that they are already in a state of oxidative stress, so the additional burden of free-radical release caused by infection overwhelms their antioxidant capacity.

Free radicals have beneficial as well as toxic effects. The phagocytes that swing into action when a pathogen breaches physical barriers release a barrage of free radicals that kill bacteria and disable viruses.[15] Moderate levels of free radicals are essential for the healing of wounds and stimulate tissue repair and regeneration.[16] However, animal and human studies have shown that the uncontrolled and excessive release of free radicals leads to organ damage, and in extreme cases, even death.

Maintaining the delicate balance between these two antagonistic actions of free radicals plays a critical role in keeping us healthy, and preventing chronic inflammation. This is where antioxidants help. Antioxidants are naturally occurring molecules that can act as an off-switch for free-radical production and compensate for many of their negative effects.

Some antioxidants are endogenous—that is, made by the body itself. Others come from food and/or supplements. One familiar endogenous antioxidant is a molecule called Coenzyme Q10 (CoQ10). All tissues require CoQ10, as it is involved in the generation of cellular energy. CoQ10 is familiar to anyone who takes cholesterol-lowering medications called "statins." Statin drugs interfere with the ability to make CoQ10, and since all cells require a constant supply of it, patients taking statins are often advised to take CoQ10 supplements.[17]

There are antioxidants that are part of our defence against oxidative stress that we cannot make ourselves. These include vitamins A, C and E, and some trace minerals like manganese, iron, selenium and zinc. All these nutrients are critical for immune functioning, and shortfalls of any one of them will compromise our ability to cope with infection.[18] In chapter 6 we will discuss whether over-the-counter supplements of vitamins and other essential nutrients could provide additional protection against inflammation, and might indeed be necessary for optimal immune support.

THE ANTI-INFLAMMATORY DIET

The anti-inflammatory diet is not a diet per se, but a way of eating designed to prevent or reduce low-grade chronic inflammation. One frequently cited anti-inflammatory diet is the Mediterranean diet, inspired by traditional eating habits of some countries around the Mediterranean Sea. The diet is rich in vegetables and fruit, herbs, spices, fish and nuts—all foods that would have been familiar to our hunter-gatherer ancestors. The Mediterranean diet has been shown to lower the risk of obesity, cancer, diabetes and heart disease and enhance life expectancy.[19]

The reason a diet rich in plant foods has such a huge role to play in protecting health is their high content of chemicals called phytochemicals. These are molecules that plants produce to protect themselves from microbial pathogens and harsh environmental conditions. Phytochemicals are powerful antibiotics, antivirals and antifungals. They are also powerful antioxidants.

Plants make the earth's atmosphere habitable for animal life by absorbing atmospheric carbon dioxide and releasing oxygen. They need some of that oxygen for their own metabolism, but it's only a fraction of what they release, so the remainder is available for our use. However, this entire process exposes plants to high levels of oxidative stress, and so they make antioxidants for their own protection.

Phytochemicals can be detected in plants because they are sensory chemicals; that is, they give colour, aroma and flavour. So, the more naturally colourful our meals, the more flavourful and aromatic they are, the greater their antioxidant content. This explains why herbs and spices, even when dried and lurking in the back of our cupboards for months, are also considered part of a nutritious diet. When we eat a plant-rich diet, we are eating an anti-inflammatory diet.

The Mediterranean diet is also high in seafood and fatty fish, which in turn is rich in essential fats called omega-3 fatty acids. Omega-3s are important components of the membranes that surround each cell. They are involved in the activation of cells from both the innate and the adaptive immune system, and they, too, are anti-inflammatory. Omega-3 fats are needed to control and subdue the excessive inflammation and release of free radicals that are the hallmark of a cytokine storm.[20]

Personally, I am particularly fond of fish, and it would be no hardship for me to eat it three times a day, seven days a week. However, our oceans are now so heavily polluted with mercury, plastics and other environmental contaminants that it is no longer considered safe to do so. In chapter 6, we will discuss safe ways of getting enough of the anti-inflammatory omega-3 fats into our diet by using supplements.

FRUITS AND VEGETABLES: HOW MUCH IS ENOUGH?

It can come as a shock to realize that for best health, we need a very high intake of phytochemical-rich vegetables and/or fruit every day—about double the five servings a day we have until recently been exhorted to eat. Multiple studies from different parts of the world have consistently shown that five servings have little or no impact on reducing the risk of cancer, heart disease or dying from any illness (all-cause mortality). But as daily intake increases to six, seven, eight, nine and then ten servings, disease risk comes down a little bit more with each additional serving.[21]

This is one area where the most recent revision of Canada's Food Guide excels, since it heavily emphasizes the need for more plants in our diet. Visit Health Canada's website and you'll see an illustration of what they call "the healthy plate," which consists of 50 per cent vegetables and/or fruit.[22] However, since the healthy plate looks very much like a dinner plate, in my experience most people take this visual to mean we need to consume lots of plant foods only at dinnertime. But in order to meet the optimal intake of ten servings a day, vegetables and/or fruit need to be a major component of each meal, not just dinner.

What is a serving size? It's a baseball-sized piece of fruit, half a cup of diced fruit or vegetables, or one whole cup of leafy greens. Initially, the idea of consuming so many vegetables every day is likely to be daunting, and it is unlikely that you'll achieve your ten-a-day goal overnight. Gradually increase your intake by replacing less nourishing, higher-calorie carbohydrate-rich foods like bread and cookies with lower-calorie, more nourishing vegetables. Remember: the more colorful you can make your meal, the more antioxidants you are eating.

Apart from its antioxidant content, there are several reasons why a plant-rich diet can help with weight control and stop us from overeating. Because of its high content of non-digestible fibre, this diet makes us feel full for longer. And at a molecular level, phytochemicals have been shown to stimulate cellular pathways involved in weight loss, an effect that appears to be comparable to restricting calories.[23] In addition, phytochemicals are natural toxins, made by the plant to ward off insect attacks and protect it from infection. Up to a certain intake, we benefit from their antioxidant and anti-infective properties. But, as the saying goes, the dose makes the poison. A very high intake eventually signals us to stop eating all those phytochemicals—before they begin to have a negative effect. So, to control inflammation and help us limit excessive food intake, vegetables are our friends!

It is important to realize that to absorb phytochemicals, they should be eaten with fat. One study looked at the absorption of the yellow/orange/red pigments of fruits and vegetables called "carotenoids," eaten as salads containing cherry tomatoes and carrots, and using either zero-fat, fat-reduced or full-fat salad dressing. With zero-fat dressing, there was no absorption at all, and only slightly more when the salad was consumed with fat-reduced dressing. A high level of absorption was seen only when full-fat salad dressing was used.[24]

So, remember to include some source of fat whenever you eat fruits or vegetables. It doesn't need to be a lot: a knob of butter or some olive oil on your vegetables, full-fat yogurt with berries, or a piece of cheese with an apple will do the job.

THE "SOUL" OF IMMUNITY

The thymus gland is a rather overlooked component of the immune network. Not to be confused with the thyroid gland, its name derives from the Greek word *thumos*, which means "soul," since the ancient Greeks believed the soul resided in the thymus. As we saw in chapter 3, the thymus is where immature lymphocytes eventually mature into fully functional T cells. The thymus is also responsible for eliminating autoreactive cells—cells that make antibodies against the body's own tissues—that may trigger autoimmune diseases.

The Greek physician Galen (circa 130–210 AD) was the first to observe that the thymus gland increases in size over the course of childhood, but after reaching peak size at about fourteen years of age, it surprisingly begins to shrink. Gradually, the active hormone-secreting cells become fewer and fewer, and are replaced by fat cells and connective tissue.

The thymus gland was thought to be of little importance until its critical role in nurturing T cells was discovered in the 1960s. In our twenties and thirties, we have an abundance of well-trained mature T cells, ready to fight off viruses and other pathogens. But by the time we are in our fifties, only about 15 per cent of active thymus tissue remains, and by the time we are in our mid-seventies, the thymus gland has dwindled to a mere shadow of its young self.

Reduction in the volume of the human thymus gland from puberty onwards continues at a rate of 3 to 5 per cent annually until middle age, when it slows down to less than 1 per cent a year. Extrapolating from this observation, scientists predict that we would totally lose thymus function at 120 years of age[25]—which, interestingly enough, is roughly the maximum human lifespan.[26]

Apart from aging, factors like smoking, alcohol and drug

abuse all prematurely age the thymus.[27] During acute infection, the thymus gland shrinks rapidly but usually recovers to its pre-infection size a few weeks after the infection resolves. This recovery may be delayed or incomplete when infectious diseases are chronic, as in HIV/AIDS.[28]

Why, as the body grows older, would an organ so critical to immunity shrink so dramatically? One explanation is that the thymus and human immunity may have evolved simply to last forty to fifty years, which for millennia was the natural maximum lifespan of most humans. And so, as medicine has advanced and life expectancy has increased, we expect our immune system to work beyond its designated lifespan.

However, there may be an alternative and more life-affirming explanation. For at least half a century, we have known that the thymus gland is exquisitely sensitive to poor nutrition. Inadequate dietary intake of protein, as well as deficiencies of key micronutrients such as zinc and antioxidant vitamins, are the main culprits. Deficiencies of any of these will cause thymic atrophy, resulting in a deficiency of the T cells that are critical for adaptive immunity.[29]

Moreover, we also know that nutritional interventions—enhanced protein intake and adequate intake of essential vitamins and minerals—can stimulate regeneration of the thymus, so that rejuvenation of the thymus may be possible.[30] This suggests that careful diets throughout our lives might extend thymus function, supporting a stronger immune system as we age.

PROTEIN, PROTEIN, PROTEIN

Protein is the main building block of the human body. Its name is derived from the Greek *protos*, meaning "first," reflecting protein's primary importance in maintaining health. Skin, nails and hair are protein. Muscles and connective tissues are protein. Protein provides the scaffolding upon which minerals are affixed to build healthy bones. Our lungs, heart, kidneys and bladder are mainly protein, as are blood and the veins and arteries that transport the blood around the body. Excluding water, our bodies are almost entirely made of protein.

Many molecules, including the hormones and neurotransmitters necessary to coordinate and regulate activity in all organs and tissues, are made from amino acids. These are the building blocks of protein, which are released when protein is digested. Key immune molecules, such as interferon, other cytokines and antibodies, are also made from amino acids. The manufacture of all these functional molecules depends on a regular supply of dietary protein.

Our bodies cannot store protein. Because we cannot function without hormones and neurotransmitters, within one to three days of not eating protein, our body will begin to break down muscle tissue to provide the amino acids it needs to survive. This is the reason why you may see visible muscle wasting after a long illness. The elderly—particularly those living alone, who may have little appetite or interest in food—frequently develop a muscle-wasting condition called sarcopenia, an age-related decrease in muscle mass which impacts strength and functioning. Protein supplementation in those at risk of sarcopenia will preserve lean body mass, and can prevent the development of frailty in the elderly.[31]

There is a process, employed by major manufacturing companies to increase efficiency and reduce costs, called "just-in-time inventory." Instead of stockpiling finished products, whether they are cars or washing machines, component parts are ordered only as needed and the finished goods are produced only when orders come in, and not before.

I find this a useful way to think of the hormones, neurotransmitters and molecules of the immune system. We don't stockpile them. When we need them, we must be able to produce them lickety-split. And to do that efficiently, we need to maintain constant blood levels of the raw materials needed for their manufacture. Those raw materials are the amino acids that come from our meal-by-meal protein intake.

HOW MUCH PROTEIN DO WE NEED?

It is often said that we eat too much protein. Certainly, in many countries, protein consumption exceeds the recommended dietary allowance (RDA). RDAs are the levels of intake of essential nutrients judged to be adequate to meet the needs of practically all healthy persons. However, RDAs represent the minimum amount needed to prevent illness, and are not necessarily optimal.

The RDA for protein is currently set at 0.8 grams per kilogram body weight per day, but many nutritional experts insist that there are specific situations where more protein may be better. Nancy Rodriguez, a professor of nutritional science at the University of Connecticut and a registered dietitian, was one of a group of sixty international scientists and nutrition experts who gathered in Washington, DC, in October 2013 to review the role of protein in health.

"There's a misunderstanding not only among the public, but also somewhat in our profession about the RDA [for protein]," she said at that time. "People in general think we all eat too much protein." On the contrary, Rodriguez added, a daily intake of protein that is twice the current RDA "is a safe and good range to aim for."[32]

If your weight creeps up even though your diet hasn't changed much, as can happen as we age, there is important recent science that may help you adjust your eating habits to make it easier to maintain a healthy BMI. Total energy expenditure (TEE) is the number of calories you burn in a day. It includes energy expended to maintain core body activities like breathing and blood circulation, the energy required to digest, absorb and store food and maintain body temperature, as well as energy used for physical activity. TEE varies a great deal from person to person. Recently, researchers have shown that a higher-protein diet also helps burn calories at a faster rate by revving up daily TEE.[33]

We know that excess calories eaten either as protein, fat or carbohydrate will be converted to fat and stored, so we must be careful to avoid overeating any of the major food groups. However, studies going back several decades have shown that replacing some dietary calories from carbohydrate with the same number of calories from protein may help you lose weight and keep it off, and also helps reduce risk of heart disease.[34]

Using new and more up-to-date methods for estimating protein needs, scientific consensus is that the current RDA for protein is too low, and that the following amounts are more likely to be optimal for daily needs.[35, 36]

For weight loss and maintenance	1.2–1.6 grams per kilogram body weight per day
For bone health and to prevent osteoporosis	1.2–1.6 grams per kilogram body weight per day
For those 65 years and older	A minimum of 1.2 grams per kilogram body weight per day
For heavy exercisers	2.0 grams per kilogram body weight per day
For surgical recovery and in intensive care	1.2–2.5 grams per kilogram body weight per day

In practice, this means that for the average 70-kilogram adult currently in good health, a daily basic minimum intake of 85–90 grams per day would be optimal.

For most people in North America, the evening meal is when most of our daily protein intake is consumed, whereas breakfast is typically carbohydrate-rich and low in protein. However, recent research has shown the importance of distributing protein intake throughout the day, not just in the elderly but in healthy adults of any age.[37] This will ensure the availability of critical amino acids all day long, not just after dinner.

MEATLESS MONDAYS

You may have heard of "meatless Mondays," and indeed, may already be including them in your weekly meal plans. The idea for meatless Mondays began in 2003 as the Monday Campaign—a non-profit organization developed in association with the John Hopkins Bloomberg School of Public Health. The message of meatless Mondays is simple: cut out meat once a week, and you not only improve your own health, but by reducing your carbon footprint, you help prevent global warming and improve the health of the planet.

It is not within the scope of this book to dissect the arguments for and against the impact of animal foods on the health of the planet, which have become heated, emotional and politicized. Suffice it to say that the jury is still out, and that some scientists calculate that the health of our planet would not be significantly improved by excluding all animal products from our diets.[38]

When the concept of meatless Mondays was first introduced, saturated fat was thought to be mainly responsible for heart disease, and was also implicated in the development of type 2 diabetes. The Monday Campaign was launched with the goal of improving heart health by reducing saturated fat intake by 15 per cent. Since animal products are the main source of saturated fat, a once-a-week meat holiday would achieve that goal. However, multiple studies have since shown that saturated fat is not responsible for the clogged arteries of heart disease. Indeed, some studies have found that saturated fat can slow the progression of existing cardiovascular disease.[39]

Now we know that both heart disease and diabetes are inflammatory processes and that the best diets to prevent them are, like the Mediterranean diet, rich in anti-inflammatory nutrients and antioxidants. If you want to prevent heart disease and diabetes, you need to ramp up your intake of vegetables and fruit, as well as good fats and oils from fish, nuts and seeds.[40]

Although plant proteins have the benefit of containing phytochemicals not found in most animal sources of protein, they either have a very low content of amino acids or lack one or two essential amino acids altogether, and so are considered incomplete. We need all the essential amino acids to build cells and maintain tissues. However, different plant foods can be mixed together to provide these—for example, eating beans and rice together will provide you with complete protein. If you are a vegan or vegetarian, you might want to talk to a dietitian to ensure your diet is providing enough complete protein.

A problem I see with meatless Mondays is that families buying into the concept often think that if avoiding meat on Mondays is good for them, it must be even better for them to extend their meat holiday to Tuesday or Wednesday or even avoid animal protein altogether. Weight for weight, animal foods provide more protein of higher quality in fewer calories than plant sources. For example, half a large chicken breast (an 85 gram serving) provides 28 grams of protein. To get the same amount of protein from cooked beans, you would need to eat 2½ cups. Such a large serving of beans would leave you feeling uncomfortably full and probably bloated.

You would also consume many more calories—850 for the beans, compared with 141 for the chicken. When substituting plant-based protein for animal sources on meatless Mondays, I find that people are either not consuming enough to provide optimal protein intake, or if they do, they are overconsuming calories and would be highly susceptible to weight gain.

Note that there are websites providing nutritional information that quote the amount of protein in beans as grams per dry weight. This can be confusing because beans are inedible unless soaked in water overnight and thoroughly cooked. The water absorbed during this process increases the weight and bulk of the beans considerably. As a rough guide, one cup of cooked beans has a protein content equivalent to 1½ ounces (45 grams) of meat or fish.

Animal-based proteins are more efficiently used by the body to build muscle and lean body mass.[41] It's not that you can't build muscle from plant-based protein. You certainly can, as vegan bodybuilders, who eat no animal foods at all, can attest. But if you're not a bodybuilder and don't expend large amounts energy through exercise, you should be aware of the high energy content in vegetarian proteins.

When we look at the guidelines for the quantity of protein that supports healthy bones, protects against weight gain and frailty and prevents loss of muscle mass with age, animal protein wins out every time.

DIABETES, SUGAR AND "NEOCARBS"

All food is made up of three main macronutrients: protein, fat and carbohydrate or "carbs." Most people understand that carbs affect your blood sugar (blood glucose) and that in those with diabetes or at risk of diabetes, blood sugar levels are too high. Persistently high circulating blood sugar, known medically as hyperglycemia, has serious health consequences. It damages the vessels that supply blood to vital organs. In turn, this increases the risk of heart disease and stroke, and induces kidney failure, nerve damage (peripheral neuropathy) and vision loss.

Hyperglycemia can significantly alter innate immune response. Dysfunction of the immune response in diabetes leads to failure to control the spread of invading pathogens, making diabetics very susceptible to infection. Even short-lived hyperglycemia can be a problem. Patients who develop stress-related hyperglycemia during a hospital stay are at increased risk of acquiring a serious infection while in hospital.[42]

The body normally controls high blood sugar levels by secreting insulin from the pancreas. Insulin helps blood sugar levels return to normal by prompting cells to absorb sugar, either for storage or for immediate use as energy. However, constant surges of insulin caused by modern diets will eventually lead to a condition known as insulin resistance, whereby cells become less sensitive to the action of insulin. Consequently, blood sugar will remain high despite adequate insulin secretion.

And it's not just sugar itself in the diet that causes high blood sugar levels. Starch is composed of long chains of sugar molecules. Although starchy foods may not taste sweet, all starch eventually digests into sugars. Eating too many starchy carbohydrates—in foods like bread, pasta, rice and potatoes—increases the risk of insulin resistance and is a known risk factor for type 2 diabetes.[43] It's OK to eat one serving of starch per meal, but don't base the meal around starches. One serving of bread is one slice; a serving of rice, potato or pasta is half a cup.

All carbs are not created equal, and some will increase blood sugar more quickly than others. The glycemic index (GI) ranks foods on a scale from 0 to 100 based on how much and how quickly they raise blood sugar after consumption. Foods with a high glycemic index, like bread, are rapidly digested. A modest intake of bread can be perfectly healthy, especially if dense and grainy and made from whole grains. But a high intake of any starchy carbohydrate causes substantial fluctuations in blood sugar and eventually leads to insulin resistance. While poor diet cannot entirely be blamed for the dramatic increase in type 2 diabetes worldwide, large-scale human studies have shown that diets based on foods with high glycemic indexes play a major role in increasing the likelihood of developing diabetes.

If you have been diagnosed with diabetes, it may seem logical to take one of the increasing number of medications now available to control blood sugar. However, a growing number of physicians worldwide are using another equally logical and drug-free approach: eliminate or drastically reduce high-GI foods that push insulin up in the first place—the sugars and starches. Eating a low-GI diet can not only control blood sugar in diabetes and prediabetes, but also reduce body weight.[44] Although this is often called low-carb eating, the term is really a misnomer, since we must not forget that vegetables and fruit are carbs, too, and as we have seen, a high intake of these plant foods is anti-inflammatory and essential for preventing diabetes.

In the UK, one doctor has found a way to help his patients understand where the hidden sugars lie in foods and how to eat in such a way that not only reduces the risk of diabetes, but can also reverse it. By following a lower carbohydrate diet, 47 per cent of diabetic and 93 per cent of prediabetic patients in his practice were able to reduce their weight, normalize blood sugar levels and reduce cholesterol and blood pressure, as well as significantly reduce the number of drugs they needed.[45]

HOW NOT TO EAT

If we do not yet have definitive answers about how to eat for the best possible health, we certainly know how *not* to eat. The Western, or standard American, diet is one of the worst in the world.

Also known appropriately by its acronym, SAD, the diet relies largely on heavily processed, factory-prepared foods.[46] It is high in processed grains and dairy, saturated and trans fats, red and processed meats, sweets and desserts, and low in fish, good fats and fruits and vegetables. The diet contains too much sodium, and way too many calories from solid fats and added sugars.

Along with a caloric intake well beyond what is necessary for most people's daily metabolic needs, the SAD diet is short of the micronutrients needed to process those calories.[47] Worldwide, every country that has adopted Western-style dietary patterns has seen an increase in obesity and diet-related chronic diseases.[48]

The good news is that by changing diets and following a healthy lifestyle, we can add as much as a decade to our lifespan.[49] While the impact of diet on aging and the prevention of chronic disease is well researched, the vital role our food plays in supporting the immune system is only now finally gaining attention. That attention is long overdue.

THE WELL-FED IMMUNE SYSTEM: SUMMARY

1. Emphasize colourful vegetables, fruits, herbs and spices. Aim for 8 to 10 servings of vegetables and fruit combined per day. Don't forget that they need to be eaten with a source of fat for optimal absorption of immune-enhancing anti-inflammatory phytochemicals.

2. Don't underestimate your daily protein needs, but remember to divide your protein intake equally between all three meals. To maintain healthy bones and for weight loss and maintenance, you need a minimum of 1.2 grams per kilogram of body weight per day.

3. To aid absorption of health-promoting phytochemicals, include a source of good fats with every meal and snack. Good fats may include olive oil, fatty fish like salmon and trout, avocados, nuts and seeds, and nut and seed butters.

4. To control weight and keep blood sugar under control, keep your meals low in high-glycemic starchy carbohydrates like bread, pasta, rice and potatoes.

5. Don't overeat, but make sure the food you do eat packs in as much nutrition as possible: focus on foods with the most nutrients that are lowest in calories—leafy green and colourful vegetables, low-calorie sources of protein and good fats with each meal.

CHAPTER SIX

Nutritional Supplements and Immunity

A vitamin is a substance that makes you ill if you don't eat it.
—Albert Szent-Györgyi, winner of the Nobel Prize
in Physiology or Medicine, 1937

As the months went by, the coronavirus originally isolated from Wuhan was mutating, although most of the changes were not seen as a cause for concern. Then, as the second wave gathered speed towards the end of the year, scientists observed a change in the spike protein—the D614G mutation—that could make COVID-19 more difficult to contain. This mutation allowed the virus to transmit slightly faster and cause larger clusters of infections.[1] Infected individuals had considerably higher viral counts in their noses and throats, and although this did not appear to make them sicker, it made it easier for them to spread the virus. Gradually, the new strain displaced earlier ones, and by December it had become the dominant strain worldwide.[2]

One concern was whether a mutation could hamper efforts to find a vaccine, since it was the original Wuhan virus that was being used as the template for vaccine development. However, most scientists felt that any mutations observed up to the end of 2020 were insufficient to endanger the effectiveness of vaccines currently in clinical trials.

But larger clusters of cases inevitably meant higher rates of hospitalization. As intensive care units filled up, doctors in many parts of the country worried that soon they would be forced to make life-or-death decisions, deciding who should have care and who should not. Some parts of Canada fared better than others. Atlantic Canada had few cases, whereas many hospitals in Manitoba, Alberta, Ontario and Quebec could hardly keep pace with the escalating number of new patients arriving daily.

In December, another mutant—B117—was identified and found to be responsible for the rapid rise in new cases in England. This variant featured multiple changes in genes that programmed the spike protein, and in one week it accounted for a doubling in the number of COVID-19 cases in and around London and southeast England. The B117 mutation made the virus as much as 70 per cent more transmissible. Again, there was no evidence that these changes jeopardized vaccine development. Although it was not clear yet if it caused more serious or fatal disease, it did spread faster, and more infection meant more opportunities for the virus to mutate, increasing the possibility that an even more virulent strain would eventually emerge.

There was concern that children were more vulnerable to the

B117 strain. "There is a hint that it has a higher propensity to infect children," said Neil Ferguson, a professor and infectious disease epidemiologist at Imperial College London. Around the world, countries closed their borders to travel from the UK. Canada suspended all flights to and from the UK on December 20. Several European countries reported the presence of the new mutation, and soon it was being picked up in Canada and the United States.

Any illusion that we had this virus under control was fading fast.

SAVE THE FRONT PAGE— THE VACCINES ARRIVE!

The delivery and distribution of the first vaccines to Canada, the UK and the United States a few weeks before Christmas provided a little distraction and a glimmer of hope. The first two vaccines to be rolled out were mRNA vaccines—quick to develop, but delicate and needing careful handling. One of them, made by Pfizer and BioNTech, needed to be maintained at minus 70 degrees Celsius, and the infrastructure to handle such cold temperatures for storage and distribution was not widely available. The other mRNA vaccine, developed in the United States by Moderna and the National Institutes of Health, was less fussy and only needed to be kept at minus 20 degrees Celsius.

Although these vaccines were the first to arrive, they were not the only ones on the horizon—at least 120 different vaccines were in clinical trials worldwide, using a variety of different delivery systems. The simultaneous exploration of different approaches to vaccine development had many advantages: if any single vaccine proved to be ineffective, there were others waiting in the wings. If, on the other hand, multiple vaccines proved effective, this would enhance capacity to produce the many billions of vaccine doses that would be needed for global distribution.

The Herculean task of manufacturing and distributing vaccines would need the cooperation of many players: governments, scientists, philanthropists and industry. The army, which is used to the deployment of troops and supplies during complex military operations, was recruited to help with vaccine distribution, especially the difficult task of getting vaccines safely to Canada's most remote and isolated communities.

Hospitals and public health officials trumpeted the arrival of the vaccines and televised the administration of the first batches. Their message was clear: we now had the tools we needed to win this war, a war with an invisible enemy, and one that some people still could not believe even existed. Despite the optimism, vaccinating a hundred thousand individuals did not put an end to the pandemic. It would likely take a year or more before mass vaccinations would be completed.

In the meantime, strict public health measures—masks, handwashing, physical distancing and avoiding large gatherings—would have to remain in place.

INFECTION SEVERITY AND IMMUNITY

It may seem reasonable to assume that those hit hardest by COVID-19 had the weakest immune systems, but this was not necessarily the case. When researchers looked for SARS-COV2-specific antibodies and T lymphocytes—two key indicators that an adequate response to the virus had occurred—they found evidence of robust responses even in the gravely ill and those who later died.[3]

If it wasn't a weaker immune system that was responsible for the most severe symptoms of COVID-19, what *was* responsible? As we have seen earlier, a disastrous overreaction of the immune system known as a "cytokine storm" appears to be the main culprit: high levels of the signalling molecules, the cytokines, that orchestrate a normal healthy immune response continue to be released long after the infection is under control. The result is an aggressive inflammatory response that can wreak widespread damage on healthy tissues.

Now blood vessels start to leak, blood pressure drops and blood clots form. Unless the inflammatory attack can be reined in, sepsis and catastrophic organ failure follows.

DRUG TREATMENT AND COVID-19

Early on in the pandemic, many different pharmaceutical treatments were tried, in the hope that an existing drug or combination of drugs might be found to help the sickest patients. Although several appeared promising at first, when tested in clinical trials, only two drugs made the cut. One was the antiviral drug Remdesivir, previously shown to have some benefit during SARS and MERS. The other was dexamethasone, a steroid with well-known immunosuppressive properties.

In keeping with what we knew about viral infections, Remdesivir was of little use if given too late in the disease. It worked best in the early stages, helping to prevent the virus from getting out of hand. But even then, it simply shortened recovery time from fifteen days to ten. It did not reduce the use of ventilators or prevent deaths. In addition to being inconvenient—it needed to be given intravenously for five days—the drug was hugely expensive: a five-day course cost over $3,200 (US). Clearly, there was a lot of money to be made during the pandemic from drugs that showed even a hint of being helpful.

Despite the hefty price tag and the limited evidence for effectiveness, in October the European Union inked an agreement with Gilead Sciences, the manufacturers of Remdesivir, to deliver a six-month supply at a cost of $1.2 billion (US). That same month, the US Food and Drug Administration (FDA) approved the use of Remdesivir in the United States—making it the first drug to receive FDA approval for COVID-19.

Scientists were baffled at the decision. Since most people recovered from the virus without any treatment, "the argument that the earlier you use it the better is great until you realize what the implications of that are," said Professor Martin Landray at the University of Oxford. "You won't save many lives, and you'll have to treat a lot of patients . . . and it'll cost a fortune."[4] Serious side effects were also showing up—in particular, kidney and liver failure—so the risk of taking the drug very likely outweighed any benefits.

The steroid drug dexamethasone fared somewhat better. It had been used for decades to calm excessive inflammation in conditions like rheumatoid arthritis and inflammatory bowel disease, as well as in intensive care units for pneumonia. It was cheap and known to be relatively safe. In patients with severe COVID-19, dexamethasone might help to dampen the excessive inflammatory response of a cytokine storm and prevent the progression of organ damage.

Initially, the World Health Organization advised against the routine use of steroids. In the early stage of an infection, a strong immune response is critical, so early treatment with immuno-suppressive drugs could be harmful, even life-threatening. However, in September they changed their minds: low doses of dexamethasone or other steroids could be helpful, they agreed, but only for patients with severe and critical COVID-19.[5] In other words, patients who had moved beyond the stage of infection control and were now suffering from their own immune system running wild.

Over the past several decades, a new discipline—nutritional immunology—has emerged that, in my opinion, has not received the attention it deserves. Nutritional immunology quite clearly shows how crucial vitamins and minerals are to a healthy immune system: they are an integral part of kick-starting the immune system into action at the first signs of infection, and then, once the infection is subdued, generous amounts are needed to scale back inflammation and prevent the immune system from going rogue.[6]

The research in this rapidly expanding field is substantial: in December 2020, a search of the scientific literature revealed over twenty-five thousand papers currently in press demonstrating links between the availability of key nutrients and a healthy immune response. The most studied include the fat-soluble vitamins A and D, the water-soluble B vitamins (folate and vitamins B_6 and B_{12}), and vitamin C, together with the minerals and trace elements magnesium, zinc and selenium.[7]

Among nutritional immunologists, there is little argument that shortages of any of these will cause immune impairment,[8] or that this immune dysregulation can be reversed by prompt and adequate supplementation.[9] So, is poor nutrition the link between chronic disease and increased susceptibility to COVID-19? Many researchers think so.[10] Underlying deficiencies of the very nutrients so vital for defence against infection are known to be common in older people,[11] in the overweight or obese[12] and in those with chronic disease.[13] It is tempting, then, to think that the shortfalls of nutrients seen in patients with conditions like diabetes, high blood pressure and heart disease are the root cause of their significantly increased risk of severe or fatal outcomes should they succumb to COVID-19.[14]

According to Health Canada, 44 per cent of adults twenty years of age and older suffer from at least one of these chronic conditions.[15] As mutations like the B117 variant increase the rate of spread of COVID-19, it's clear that the high incidence of chronic disease, in Canada and in all developed nations, puts not just the elderly at risk of severe or fatal disease, but large swaths of younger populations as well.

ARE RECOMMENDED DAILY INTAKES ADEQUATE?

The establishment of recommended nutrient intakes began in the United States around 1940. The Second World War had resulted in serious malnutrition in many parts of Europe. To ensure that the food rations sent to American troops fighting in Europe were nutritionally adequate, desirable levels of protein, energy and eight vitamins and minerals were established. The recommendations were subsequently adopted by Canada and the UK. These early guidelines were thought to be sufficient to prevent any of the deficiency diseases known at the time, such as scurvy, an indicator of serious vitamin C deficiency.[16]

Theoretically, it's impossible to be deficient in an essential nutrient and survive. They are, after all, *essential*—in other words, necessary for all life processes to continue. Although vitamins and minerals—the micronutrients—are needed only in tiny amounts compared to fat, protein and carbohydrate, getting too little of any one of them can have devastating consequences. As researchers like Sir Robert McCarrison discovered early in the twentieth century: deprive an animal of any one of these critical dietary elements for long enough, and that animal will die.

The intakes of vitamins officially recommended were just sufficient to prevent physical signs of deficiency in most of the population, plus a little extra to cover individual variations in needs. But even in the early days of developing recommendations, it was acknowledged that improvement in the growth and functioning of animals, including humans, could be seen when intakes were increased beyond the basic requirements. However, no attempt was made to define *optimal* intakes—amounts that would sustain all body tissues and organs in good health.[17]

In 1989, the number of vitamins and minerals with recommended daily intakes increased from the original eight to twenty-five, as knowledge grew about other vitamins and nutrients and their deficiency diseases.

RECOMMENDED INTAKES DO NOT
MEET TODAY'S NEEDS

Towards the end of the twentieth century, it was gradually acknowledged that we had a problem with current recommendations. Good nutrition should do more than just prevent signs of deficiencies; it should support robust good health. Daily recommended intakes (DRIs) for nutrients, it was concluded, might be enough to prevent frank deficiency diseases, but they were insufficient to head off chronic diseases.

Chronic diseases do not necessarily exhibit classical signs of deficiency, but they do involve tissue deterioration and a breakdown of innate abilities to control vital body processes like blood pressure or blood glucose. Based on current evidence, nutritional immunologists believe that intakes above currently recommended levels will be needed to optimize immune responses and increase resistance to infection.[18]

From November 2014 until April 2016, a working group sponsored by the Canadian and US governments met to see if they could establish reference values appropriate for preventing such conditions as diabetes and cardiovascular disease and establish a Chronic Disease Risk Reduction Intake (CDRR).[19] After five years of deliberation, the working group had prioritized sodium, potassium, the omega-3 fatty acids, vitamin E and magnesium for further review. To date, CDRRs have been established only for sodium and potassium.[20] We still have no recommendations for amounts of other nutrients that might be optimal for chronic disease prevention. For example, magnesium deficiency is a major global concern and a risk factor for cardiovascular disease.[21] While it is known that the majority of North Americans do not meet current DRIs for magnesium, we still have no idea whether the DRI is sufficient or an even higher intake of magnesium would be needed to prevent high blood pressure, irregular heartbeats or heart attacks, all of which are linked to magnesium deficiency.[22]

Apart from the handful of nutrients already earmarked for consideration, the other vitamins and minerals aren't even on the radar screen for review. But the committee has admitted that the task they have been given is a difficult one—one that is much more difficult than originally believed. Chronic diseases are complex and involve shortfalls of more than one nutrient and risk factors other than nutrition, such as smoking and sedentary lifestyles. They are also linked to environmental and workplace exposures to toxins and pollution.[23]

Science hasn't yet come up with accurate methods for measuring such complexity, and perhaps it never will. In any event, it is clear that at the current rate of progress it is likely to be decades before Chronic Disease Risk Reduction Intakes are reviewed and set for the full range of vitamins and minerals.

During the first year of the pandemic, the pace of scientific publishing accelerated dramatically in response to the need for scientists and clinicians to share their ideas and experiences treating this virus for which there was no existing road map. Journals rushed articles into print, often with minimal peer review. Doctors were eager to share their ideas and experiences on anything and everything that might be helpful in controlling and treating the virus.

The potential for nutritional supplements to be beneficial, however, hardly got a mention: of more than eighty-six thousand papers on COVID published by the end of 2020, a mere handful—less than 1 per cent—related to vitamins, and only seven of these involved clinical trials. This was in spite of the fact that past research had repeatedly demonstrated a role for vitamin and mineral therapy in dampening the severity of upper respiratory tract infections, including pneumonia.[24] Nutrition was clearly not front-of-mind for clinicians.

It was therefore disappointing, but not surprising, that the well-established role of high-dose intravenous vitamin C (ascorbic acid) in treating sepsis and severe respiratory infection received so little attention from clinicians during the pandemic. When it is given intravenously, higher blood levels of vitamin C can be achieved compared to taking oral supplements. In general, vitamin C appears to normalize cytokine generation.[25]

Perhaps one of the most misunderstood of all the vitamins, controversy has swirled around the role of vitamin C in immunity ever since 1977, when two-time Nobel Prize winner Linus Pauling published his book *Vitamin C, the Common Cold and the Flu*, in which he suggested that daily intakes of between 200 and 3,000 milligrams of vitamin C would prevent most seasonal colds.[26] Despite Pauling's fame as a brilliant chemist and molecular biologist, the medical establishment took a very dim view of his ideas on nutrition.

There were scathing reviews of Pauling's book in medical journals—the *Journal of the American Medical Association* dismissed it as "irritating." Pauling himself readily admitted that he didn't know exactly *how* vitamin C helped control viral infections, but said, "I have, however, formulated the hypothesis that the effectiveness of ascorbic acid in providing protection against viral diseases results from its function in the synthesis and activity of interferon in preventing the entry of virus particles into the cells."[27]

As we have seen, "interferon" is actually a group of molecules that control both innate and adaptive antiviral responses and are pivotal in controlling the outcome of viral infections.[28] Interferons are the emergency flares discharged by macrophages and virally infected cells in the early stages of infection, alerting the immune network that an invasion has taken place. Be ready, they say, to marshal the troops.

Animal studies have shown that without vitamin C, interferon production ceases and viral infections becomes lethal.[29] In scurvy, the lethal disease caused by vitamin C deficiency, lung infections and pneumonia are the main cause of death. Pauling's hunch, in good part, had been right.

HIGH-DOSE INTRAVENOUS VITAMIN C AND COVID-19

Despite routinely receiving 125 milligrams of vitamin C daily, which is higher than the recommended daily intake (90 milligrams for men; 75 milligrams for women), many patients in intensive care units who are suffering from sepsis have very low or undetectable blood levels of vitamin C—an indicator of scurvy.[30]

Vitamin C not only enhances immune function, but is an important antioxidant, calming oxidative stress and reducing inflammation. Vitamin C is needed for the production of collagen, the second-most-abundant molecule in the body, after water. Collagen is the glue that holds connective tissue together. It is essential for wound healing—the complex and dynamic process of replacing destroyed and damaged tissue with healthy new tissue.

One concern that arose during the COVID-19 pandemic was the degree of scarring of organs seen in recovered patients. Called "fibrosis," this scarring reduces the flexibility of tissues and organs, interfering with their function. A fibrotic heart, for instance, cannot contract and relax properly, and fibrotic lungs don't fully expand during breathing. Vitamin C, either alone or in combination with vitamin E, can prevent experimental lung fibrosis.[31]

Multiple clinical trials have demonstrated the safety of intravenous high-dose vitamin C (between 6 and 24 grams per day) for severe respiratory infections, and results include lower mortality rates, fewer ICU and hospital stays, and less time on mechanical ventilators for patients who need them.[32] Several clinical trials of intravenous vitamin C in severely ill COVID-19 patients are underway in China, the results of which may be available soon.[33]

At Sunnybrook Hospital in Toronto and Sherbrooke University in Quebec, the LOVIT (Lessening Organ Dysfunction with Vitamin C) trial is examining whether high-dose intravenous vitamin C (50 milligrams per kilogram, every six hours for ninety-six hours) can reduce organ dysfunction in ICU patients with sepsis. This trial began recruiting patients with sepsis at twenty-five Canadian ICUs long before COVID-19 emerged in Canada, but when the WHO listed vitamin C as one of its research priorities during the pandemic, researchers modified their trial to include COVID-19 patients. The trial is ongoing and aims to recruit eight hundred patients, some of whom will be given high-dose vitamin C twice a day for four days while others receive a placebo.

While the careful investigation into the effectiveness of drugs in placebo-controlled clinical trials is always warranted before recommending their widespread use, such an approach for essential nutrients is ethically questionable. Why would you knowingly withhold vitamin C from a patient in an ICU whom you knew to have vitamin C blood levels indicative of scurvy, as seen in many—if not most—patients with sepsis?[34] Not only is vitamin

C essential for a fully functional immune system, but untreated scurvy is invariably fatal.

Because of its excellent safety record, a strong rationale for its use and sufficient preliminary data that it is effective in treating serious infections of the upper respiratory tract, intravenous vitamin C has been suggested as an obvious pragmatic approach to therapy in severe COVID-19 cases, either alone or in combination with other immune-enhancing vitamins.[35]

At the very least, it would seem obligatory to give severely ill COVID-19 patients a fighting chance by administering sufficient vitamin C to restore their blood levels to normal. Anything less seems either like wilful neglect or a basic lack of understanding of the essential nature of nutrients like vitamin C.

DO UNDERNOURISHED HOSTS DRIVE VIRAL MUTATIONS?

Are all viral mutations simply random events, or are there certain conditions or situations that increase their likelihood? Ultraviolet radiation from the sun can certainly cause multiple changes to the genetic material of viruses. However, solar radiation is also a major germicide, so it is more likely to deactivate viruses than it is to contribute to mutations.[36]

Traditionally, the nutritional status of the host was believed simply to influence their ability to respond appropriately to infection, but it is also known to alter the genetic makeup of viruses, triggering mutations.[37] In one experiment, researchers fed one group of mice a normal diet, while giving a second group a diet with insufficient selenium—a trace mineral that is a powerful antioxidant. Then the mice were infected with a mild strain of a human influenza virus.

Both groups of mice became infected, but those fed complete diets recovered quickly, while the selenium-deficient mice developed severe long-lasting infections. The scientists noted that the difference between the two groups was comparable to mild pneumonia in the well-fed group, but severe, life-threatening pneumonia in the selenium-deficient mice.[38]

In addition, the virus the researchers recovered from the selenium-deficient mice had mutated to become more virulent, whereas in animals fed a normal diet, it was unchanged. And once the virus had mutated, it could produce more severe disease even in healthy mice fed a normal diet. "These results represent a new paradigm for the interaction between host nutritional status and the emergence of new viral diseases," commented the researchers, pointing out that widespread nutritional deficiencies are common in many developing countries where new viral diseases frequently surface. "Adequate nutrition of the population is an important form of protection against the emergence of new viral pathogens," they concluded.[39]

So far, the researchers have studied only selenium and vitamin E. Deficiencies of either of these will trigger viral mutations that allow a virus to cause more severe illness in well-nourished animals. But it's likely that host deficiencies of many other nutrients

The Well-Fed Immune System

will be shown to have similar effects when investigated. Inadequate intakes of a range of micronutrients are linked to increases in oxidative stress and excessive free radical release, and consequently, DNA and RNA damage—ideal conditions to drive viral mutations.[40]

SHOULD YOU TAKE SUPPLEMENTS?

To decrease the risk of developing COVID-19 or passing it on, medical officers of health and infectious disease experts were constantly urging us to wear face masks, wash our hands regularly and practise social distancing. But unlike in some other countries, there was no mention that including a daily vitamin D supplement could complement these measures and help lower the risk of hospitalization and severe disease. The official line on vitamins was to "eat a good diet." This, we are assured, would provide us with all the micronutrients the immune system needed.

However, all the evidence pointed to the contrary. Low vitamin D status is a global health problem, not only in housebound older individuals, but in all age groups, even in geographical areas where it is possible to have year-round exposure to the sun.[41] Very few foods contain vitamin D naturally, although some foods, like milk, are fortified with vitamin D. But you would have to drink ten glasses of milk to get 1,000 international units (IU) or 25 micrograms (mcg) of vitamin D—the usual amount in one small vitamin D capsule.

On December 7, 2020, an international group of over one hundred scientists, doctors and leading authorities on vitamin D signed a letter calling on governments, public health officials, doctors and health-care workers everywhere to act immediately to recommend increased vitamin D intakes in the general population. "The preponderance of evidence indicates that increased vitamin D would help reduce infections, hospitalizations, ICU admissions and deaths," the letter stated.

In the elderly and in those with chronic diseases[42] who are at high risk of more serious symptoms if they acquire COVID-19, low blood levels of vitamins A, C, D, E and the B vitamin folate are common. In older people, these deficiencies are associated with increased frailty.[43] As we have already seen, the key nutrients we need for effective immune responses are the very ones that have been shown to be deficient in those with common chronic diseases.

We don't know for sure whether the observed deficiencies are a consequence or a cause of the chronic diseases, but there is some evidence to suggest that it may be a bit of both. For example, the chronic levels of inflammation seen in type 2 diabetes can be mitigated by the anti-inflammatory effect of vitamin C.[44] At the same time, multiple studies have shown that vitamin C supplements can control the high levels of blood glucose that cause diabetes in the first place. One study found that taking 1,000 milligrams of vitamin C a day—but not 500 milligrams—lowered elevated blood sugar into the normal range.[45] Since diabetics do not appear to have lower dietary intakes of vitamin C, it has therefore been suggested that vitamin C supplements may protect against the development of type 2 diabetes.[46]

Even in those currently free of chronic disease, less-than-optimal intakes of vitamins and other essential nutrients have consequences and increase susceptibility to future disease.[47] Nearly eighty years ago, early vitamin researchers warned of this possibility. "The majority of the public are content to spend their lives in that shadowed region between good health and frank illness. There is a wide gap between the minimum diet, which just prevents deficiency symptoms, and the optimum to promote good health. Subnormal nutrition may be present, even when there are no obvious clinical signs," wrote the editors of the textbook *The Vitamins in Medicine*, published in 1942.[48]

It is beyond the scope of this book to go into the details of how each essential nutrient impacts specific functional pathways of the immune response network. For those who want to explore molecular and biochemical interactions in more depth, there are many excellent up-to-date reviews available on nutrient-immune interactions.[49, 50]

SAFETY FIRST

Do a quick Google search, and you will encounter article after article warning of serious concerns about vitamin safety. Reading some of these articles, you might be forgiven for thinking there was growing evidence that nutritional supplements are dangerous and can cause serious health problems, even death.

Safety is, of course, a major concern and should always be a priority when considering taking supplements. But the safety record of vitamins and mineral supplements is excellent, especially when compared to the drugs—even those available over-the-counter—that millions of people take every day. One Canadian study found that one in nine patients attending hospital emergency departments was there because of an adverse reaction to a medication, even though they were taking the drug as prescribed. Of these reactions, 75 per cent were considered moderate or severe.[51]

The same is not true for vitamins and minerals. Public records show that very few deaths or serious adverse events have ever been linked to vitamins, provided they are taken as indicated on the bottle or as advised by a reputable health practitioner. However, some multivitamins or iron pills are sugar-coated and may seem like candy to a small child. Toddlers have, unfortunately, died after consuming toxic amounts of iron from adult multivitamins or iron supplements.

But this is a preventable accident, not an adverse effect.

GENES AND NUTRIENTS

When discussing adverse events in the context of nutritional supplements, we must be careful to distinguish between symptoms that cause genuine health problems and those that are merely a nuisance. For example, excess vitamin C intake from supplements can cause diarrhea. Is this an adverse effect, or is it telling us something important about our genetic makeup?

The relatively new science of nutrigenetics has shown how basic needs for vitamins can vary considerably from one person to another, depending on our genes. If you are someone with lower genetic needs for vitamin C, and you take more than you need, you might get diarrhea. This is inconvenient, but not dangerous—the body is simply eliminating excess. Just cutting back a little on your intake can eliminate this unwanted effect.

But many people will benefit from and tolerate much higher doses, especially if they lead stressful lives, since stress seriously depletes vitamin C. Personalized nutrition, sometimes called precision nutrition, is a practical approach to identifying individual genetic needs. Some nutritionally oriented doctors use a concept called "bowel tolerance" to customize vitamin C recommendations. They suggest increasing vitamin C in small doses until you do get loose stools, and then scaling back the dose slightly. Bowel tolerance for vitamin C is therefore the maximum anyone can tolerate without getting diarrhea.[52]

SUPPLEMENTS FOR IMMUNE SUPPORT

In the absence of public health direction, what can we do as individuals to safeguard our immune health? The threat facing us is immediate—we cannot wait to see what advice we eventually get on Chronic Disease Risk Reduction Intake levels, and an increasing number of research findings suggest that current daily intake recommendations are likely to be inadequate for effective immune responses in the face of a pandemic.

Should we design our own programs of supplements? If so, what doses should we use to ensure that any program we devise is helpful and unlikely to be harmful? One approach might be to aim for the Tolerable Upper Intake Level (UL), at least for those nutrients known to be needed for optimal immunity.

The ULs reflect the maximum daily intake levels at which no risk of adverse health effects is expected for almost all individuals in the general population—including sensitive ones—when a supplement is consumed over long periods of time. These levels can be used to optimize your regime and are considered appropriate for immune support and reduced risk of serious viral infections.[53] We can take the UL of a nutrient with a high degree of confidence that we will not be harmed.

For some nutrients, like vitamin B_{12} and vitamin K, there is no UL, since there is no evidence they are toxic. As the US Office of Dietary Supplements says, "no adverse effects associated with vitamin K consumption from food or supplements have been reported in humans or animals."[54] The same applies to B_{12}: in healthy people, no toxic effects have been associated with high intakes.[55]

We don't necessarily want excessive amounts: the goal is to achieve optimal intakes and a proper balance of nutrients. A balanced regime will include a range of nutrients that work together. For example, vitamin D is dependent on magnesium for its metabolism, and since magnesium deficiency is very common in North America, taking vitamin D without magnesium may not give you the benefits you expect. Do not exceed ULs unless on the advice of a knowledgeable health practitioner.

RECOMMENDATIONS

In my practice, a basic supplement regime usually includes a multivitamin, additional vitamins C, D and E, and magnesium plus omega-3 fats (fish oil). Some factors to consider when taking these supplements are considered below.

Although there are very few dangerous interactions between drugs and nutrients, there are some. For example, vitamin K interferes with the action of the drug warfarin, while birth control pills deplete many of the B vitamins. However, since most drugs have not been tested for potential interactions with nutrients, as a general rule you should allow at least two hours between taking medications and consuming supplements.

Multivitamins

If you take nothing else on a daily basis, a well-formulated multivitamin should be your first choice. A multivitamin will contain a little bit of most vitamins and minerals, and can be a useful insurance policy against nutritional gaps. Remember, no nutrient works alone. Each one depends on a host of other nutrients to work effectively and efficiently. In North America, dietary assessments repeatedly show inadequate intakes of the vitamins and minerals the immune system needs,[56] and a multivitamin will go some way towards redressing these shortfalls.

Choose a product that contains the widest spectrum of trace minerals. A good multivitamin for immune support will contain 15 milligrams of zinc, 1 milligram of copper and 100 micrograms of selenium. A multivitamin should provide a range of B vitamins, which work together and should be taken together. Since the need for B vitamins probably far exceeds the recommended daily intakes (RDI),[57] choose a multivitamin containing at least 25 milligrams of most of the B vitamins and 400 micrograms of folic acid.

Many multivitamins offer different formulations for men and women and for those over fifty years of age, so choose one appropriate for your sex and life stage. Multivitamins rarely contain enough magnesium or vitamin C or D. You will need to supplement these nutrients separately.

SPECIAL CONSIDERATIONS: Occasionally, one of the B vitamins, B_3 (niacin), will cause what is called a "niacin flush." This can appear as blotchy red patches on the skin that could be mistaken for an allergic reaction, but it is not. It usually lasts about twenty minutes and is harmless. Multivitamins have been shown to be very safe, even when taken over long periods of time.[58]

Vitamin C

As already discussed, vitamin C's antioxidant, anti-inflammatory and immunomodulating effects make it a powerful potential candidate in the prevention of infection and enhanced immune responses in COVID-19 infection.

For oral supplementation, the upper limit of vitamin C is 2 grams a day for adults. I generally suggest taking 1 gram twice a day (1 gram = 1,000 milligrams). There is a threshold for absorbing vitamin C. Doses between 200 and 400 milligrams are well absorbed, but intakes beyond that will generally be rapidly excreted in urine.

Since vitamin C is constantly being depleted by stress, I recommend taking time-released forms of vitamin C. These are formulated to gradually release small amounts of vitamin C over a prolonged period—usually twelve hours. Taken in the morning, time-released vitamin C will help you deal with daytime stress. But since you manufacture and repair collagen when you are asleep, a second dose later in the day is also recommended.

SPECIAL CONSIDERATIONS: Supplemental vitamin C increases output of oxalate in urine (as do spinach, coffee and tea). Theoretically, this could lead to the formation of calcium oxalate kidney stones. Massive doses of vitamin C given intravenously have not been shown to cause a problem in people with normal kidney function.[59] Nevertheless, if you have a history of kidney stone formation, you may want to consider avoiding more than 1 gram of vitamin C a day. Instead, take 500 milligrams morning and evening.

Vitamin D

We make vitamin D when we are exposed to summer sunshine. Living in northerly countries—latitudes 40 degrees north and higher—during the winter months puts everyone at risk of vitamin D deficiency. In these regions, vitamin D deficiency is especially common in the elderly, but can also affect younger age groups, especially anyone who is housebound, wears sunblock or covers up extensively while outdoors. Vitamin D recommendations are expressed in either international units or micrograms. It has been estimated that we make 10,000–25,000 IUs of vitamin D after sun exposure that produces a faint pinkness in our skin twenty-four hours later.[60] But we never get toxic from too much sun: sunshine stimulates the production of enzymes that will break down any excess vitamin D beyond a certain blood level.

Vitamin D deficiency is linked to increased risk of acquiring COVID-19 and to worse outcomes. The vitamin strengthens physical barriers against viral infections and, like vitamin C, stimulates the production of interferon—first-line defences against pathogens. By controlling the production of inflammatory cytokines, vitamin D plays a critical role in preventing a cytokine storm.[61]

Compared with light-skinned people, those with dark skin need much longer exposure to sunlight to produce equivalent amounts of vitamin D and are therefore particularly at risk of vitamin D deficiency. Since dark-skinned individuals are disproportionately affected by COVID-19 and have poorer outcomes compared to those with lighter skin, they should be particularly careful to supplement with vitamin D.

The upper limit of vitamin D is 4,000 IU per day (or 100 mcg) for those nine years and older. Some people may need more than this to raise their blood level to the top end of the normal range, which some experts believe is optimal, since it is a level that can be easily achieved by natural sun exposure in people who get reasonable amounts of sunshine all year round.[62]

If you get your blood tested, wait until three months after you start taking the UL for vitamin D. And only test in the winter, not the height of summer, when it may be temporarily high. If you have taken a sunshine holiday, wait eight weeks before testing blood levels. Take sufficient vitamin D to achieve a blood level of 175–200 nanomoles per litre (nmol/L)—or, in the United States, 80–100 nanograms per millilitre (ng/mL). Vitamin D is a fat-soluble vitamin and must be taken with food for proper absorption.

SPECIAL CONSIDERATIONS: Those who are overweight or obese generally have lower blood levels of vitamin D compared to normal-weight individuals and may need to take more vitamin D to achieve similar blood levels.[63]

Vitamin E

Vitamin E is a powerful fat-soluble antioxidant found in high concentration in immune cells. Supplementing above current dietary recommendations has been shown to enhance immunity and reduce risk of infection, particularly in older individuals.[64] Vitamin E interacts synergistically with vitamin C, so that when the two vitamins are taken together, higher blood levels of vitamin C are achieved. Conversely, higher blood levels of vitamin E are seen when it is taken with vitamin C.[65]

In nature, vitamin E occurs in eight different forms: alpha-, beta-, gamma- and delta-tocopherol and alpha-, beta-, gamma- and delta-tocotrienol. Each of these different forms of vitamin E acts as an antioxidant, but individual forms may act distinctly from one another. The UL for vitamin E has been set for alpha-tocopherol only and is 670 IU. Make sure the vitamin E you take is full spectrum—that is, it contains all eight forms of vitamin E that are naturally present in food.

Avoid synthetic versions of vitamin E (such as dl-alpha tocopherol), although you can ignore the tiny amount that may be present in a multivitamin. Capsules vary in strength from approximately 200 to 400 IU daily. For most adults, I recommend 400 IU a day. Because vitamin E is fat soluble, it needs to be taken with a meal for proper absorption.

Magnesium

As we have seen in chapter 4, magnesium is one of the trickiest nutrients to supplement, especially because of its intimate relationship with stress. Stress is known to increase magnesium loss and cause deficiency. In turn, magnesium deficiency enhances susceptibility to stress, resulting in a vicious cycle that makes maintaining consistent magnesium stores difficult.[66]

The possibility that magnesium might help in the prevention and treatment of COVID-19 has been suggested, based on its known requirement for lung function and its powerful anti-inflammatory effects.[67] We have seen that blood tests are not reliable indicators of adequate magnesium tissue stores. However, low tissue stores cause obvious physical symptoms, which include headaches and insomnia, foot or leg cramps, tremors and vertigo.

Cardiovascular symptoms include palpitations, arrhythmias and high blood pressure. In the gastrointestinal tract, low magnesium may cause reflux and constipation.[68] In someone short of magnesium, I expect to see a number of these symptoms, and when magnesium deficiency is corrected, to see most of them resolve.

The UL for magnesium is 420 milligrams for men and 320 milligrams for women. In practice, this may be too much for some and not enough for others, especially those taking medications that severely deplete magnesium, such as diuretics or anti-reflux drugs called proton pump inhibitors. Magnesium relaxes muscles, and too much magnesium will over-relax the smooth muscle of the colon, causing loose bowels. Constipation, on the other hand, is usually a sign of too little magnesium.[69]

You can personalize your magnesium intake using the bowel tolerance method described for vitamin C, but you can't use the method for both vitamin C and magnesium, so I prefer to reserve this approach for magnesium. The form of magnesium you take is important. I recommend using magnesium glycinate, which is well absorbed. Start with 100 milligrams at night, before bed. After three days, begin to slowly increase the daily dose—by 50 milligrams every three days. Alternate additions between mornings and evenings, until one to three soft, comfortable bowel movements are achieved each day.

The amount of magnesium tolerated will vary from one person to another; for some, 100 milligrams before bed may be enough, but others may tolerate 300 or 400 milligrams twice a day to achieve bowel tolerance, especially if constipation has been a problem or if they take medications that deplete magnesium. Rarely, some individuals may need even more, but high doses should be taken under the supervision of a knowledgeable health practitioner. If stools become loose, cut back daily magnesium intake by 50 milligrams.

Zinc

Zinc is required for optimal innate immune responses. Zinc deficiency affects our ability to taste and smell things normally. It is interesting that one of the symptoms now recognized as a clue that someone may test positive for COVID-19 is loss of the senses of smell and taste. If you are taking a multivitamin, it will usually contain between 10 and 15 milligrams of zinc, and for most people, this may be enough for regular use. However, during active infection, extra zinc is frequently required.

Zinc supplements have been shown to reduce the symptoms and duration of colds, which are often caused by coronaviruses, so supplementing could be helpful for COVID-19, too. Sucking low-dose zinc lozenges (8–10 milligrams each) up to a total daily dose of 80 milligrams has been shown to shorten the duration of sore throats and colds.

However, for some people, 80 milligrams might be a bit too much. Luckily, there are ways to tell when you are taking too much zinc. Most zinc lozenges have some strong flavouring, like licorice or elderberry, added. As you start to take them, they taste good. But as you take more, they may begin to taste unpleasantly metallic. This is your sign to stop taking the lozenges for that day. Resume taking them the next day, but make sure to stop when they begin to taste bad again. Regardless of how they taste, stick to a maximum of 80 milligrams of extra zinc per day (not counting what may be in your multivitamin).

SPECIAL CONSIDERATIONS: One sign of ongoing poor zinc status is the presence of little white flecks on your fingernails, known medically as leukonychia. If your nails have these, you definitely need more zinc. If you already take a multivitamin and still have leukonychia, don't wait to get sick; start taking an extra 25 milligrams of zinc daily. Because taking extra zinc can cause a relative deficiency of copper, some zinc supplements contain copper. But a multivitamin and mineral supplement containing copper will probably supply all you need.

OTHER SUPPLEMENTS TO CONSIDER

Omega-3 Fats (Fish Oil)

One of two types of essential fats, omega-3 fats are a critical component of the cell membranes of all immune cells, and they exert major changes in the activation of cells of both the innate and adaptive immune systems. Human beings are believed to have evolved on a one-to-one ratio of omega-6 to omega-3 fats, whereas in today's Western diets, the ratio is between fifteen and seventeen to one.

Excessive amounts of omega-6 fats promote inflammation,

and correcting this imbalance by consuming more omega-3 fats can suppresses inflammation.[70] Supplementing with omega-3 fats could therefore play an important role in reducing the risk of many chronic diseases. Studies show a ratio of between two and three to one suppressed inflammation in rheumatoid arthritis. A ratio of five to one was beneficial for patients with asthma, whereas a ratio of ten to one had adverse consequences.[71] In patients with severe upper respiratory tract infections given supplements of omega-3 fats in ICU, a reduction in time spent on a ventilators and fatalities was observed.[72]

The omega-6 fats are rich in vegetable and seed oils like soy, corn, safflower and sunflower oil. Omega-3 fats are mainly from fish, particularly fatty cold-water fish like salmon and trout. While fish is an excellent addition to the diet, eating too much of it has become a hazard today because of contamination with mercury and other pollutants that fish have absorbed from our deteriorating oceans. Fish oil supplements are screened for such pollution and guaranteed pure. They are therefore the safest way to consume anti-inflammatory levels of omega-3 fats.

Today's fish oil is much more pleasant to take than the cod liver oil we detested as children. Different brands vary in their concentration of the two important long-chain fatty acids—EPA and DHA. Aim for a daily dose of approximately 500 milligrams of DHA and 750 milligrams of EPA.

SPECIAL CONSIDERATIONS: A vegan diet is particularly short of omega-3 fats, so vegetarians and vegans should take omega-3 fat supplements. Algal oil made from microscopic plant forms in oceans is certified vegan-friendly.

Vitamin A

Vitamin A is found in foods from animal sources, including dairy products, fish and meat (especially liver). In the past, when we supplemented with cod liver oil, we got not only vitamin D but also vitamin A and omega-3 fats. Some plant pigments—the carotenoids—are known as provitamin A because we can convert them into vitamin A, although not very efficiently. Vegetarians can get vitamin A by consuming lots of yellow, red and orange fruits and vegetables.

Vitamin A is needed for immune cell maturation and function. In the lungs, vitamin A is needed for the maintenance of the alveoli (the air sacs where the lungs and blood exchange oxygen and carbon dioxide) and for them to regenerate after they have been damaged.[73] Chronic vitamin A deficiency can make an individual more susceptible to respiratory disease and a range of infections.

It is important to be aware that vitamin A deficiency may handicap the body's response to vaccination, reducing the level of protection achieved.[74] The Upper Tolerable Limit is 10,000 IU daily.

Vitamin K: Indispensable Companion to Vitamin D

Vitamin D and vitamin K work together and are often found together in the same supplement. Vitamin K is actually a group of vitamins, the most prominent being K_1 and K_2. Vitamin K_1 is found in green vegetables like broccoli and spinach. Certain bacteria can synthesize vitamin K_2, and it is found in fermented food like cheese and sauerkraut. Vitamin K_1 and K_2 play very similar roles in the body, but K_2 stays longer in the blood and is therefore usually used in supplements.

While vitamin D is needed to absorb calcium, vitamin K is required to bind the calcium to bones, so these vitamins work together to prevent osteoporosis. Vitamin K is also needed to block the accumulation of calcium in places where it doesn't belong, such as in blood vessel walls or in kidneys. No UL has been set for vitamin K, and no adverse effects have ever been reported.[75]

Vitamin K is essential for normal blood clotting (coagulation). It is needed to clot blood and stop bleeding. It also has opposing effects, helping to produce proteins that stop the formation of blood clots (thrombosis) in blood vessels. In severe cases of COVID-19, patients may suffer from blood clots in the legs and lungs, and from stroke-causing clots that block blood vessels supplying blood to the brain. Some researchers suspect that these blood clots may be due to vitamin K deficiency and that vitamin K might prevent the formation of thrombosis, although so far, no clinical trial have been carried out.[76]

SPECIAL CONSIDERATIONS: If you are taking blood-thinning medications, consult your doctors before taking vitamin K. Some blood thinners work by blocking the action of vitamin K, so taking it may reduce their effectiveness.

DISINFORMATION AND MISINFORMATION

Make sure that anything you are reading about supplements is from a trusted source. As in any crisis, there are always unscrupulous people seeking to exploit our anxiety to sell us products that may be worthless, using unsubstantiated health claims. The COVID-19 pandemic is no exception: a barrage of half-baked theories, vague unproven folk remedies and, unfortunately, intentionally misleading "fake news" has flooded the internet. As fast as the virus is spreading, misinformation and disinformation has spread even faster.

Be aware that some widely shared myths about the dangers of vitamins or their lack of effectiveness may come from academics, some of whom, on the face of it, should be reliable sources of information. These are the professional debunkers who make careers out of challenging popularly held beliefs, and they are the darlings of the media. However, they rarely understand nutrition in sufficient depth to be able to identify reliable research and discard the bad stuff.

After starting a supplement regime, try to take it consistently for at least a year. Then re-evaluate. Some of the benefits of supplements are subtle at first, and not everyone will experience dramatic responses immediately. You be the judge as to whether you have experienced any benefits. Has your energy increased, or your exercise tolerance improved? Are you sleeping better? Do you feel happier and more relaxed? These changes are often the first you may notice.

Does your skin look healthier? Is your hair thicker and shinier? Are your nails stronger? Expect changes like these to take a bit longer—it takes six months for a nail to grow from base to tip, so don't expect nails to stop peeling or breaking right away. Perhaps other family members have sniffled and coughed intermittently throughout the winter, but you have survived without a cold. If you would normally have a seasonal cold or two, and a year has passed during which you have been cold-free, your immune system is demonstrably better nourished.

But remember, supplements are well named—they *supplement* a good diet. They should never be used simply to compensate for poor eating habits.

Looking Back; Thinking Forward

The COVID-19 pandemic has forced many people to shelter in their homes, reduce contacts, and limit all those activities that seemed essential for their daily happiness. The world has shrunk into a small place defined by the confines of our house. Time has assumed a new dimension and seems suspended.
—The Lancet Infectious Diseases, *January 1, 2021*

It's New Year's Eve 2020. The second wave of the pandemic is in full flood. Worldwide, over one hundred million cases of COVID-19 have been confirmed, with over two million deaths. This year there will be no parties, no fireworks, no visits with friends and neighbours to clink glasses and share our hopes and ambitions for the coming year. Toronto is again in lockdown.

Following a period of relative calm over the summer when infection rates dropped—in some places to almost negligible numbers—it seemed the end of the pandemic might be in sight.

But as restrictions were relaxed and winter set in, the virus came roaring back, this time armed with a few new tricks to help it spread faster, easier. The alarming increase in infections meant more hospitalizations and fatalities. But, critically, the additional number of new infections gave the virus unlimited opportunities to mutate.

While most mutations would not favour the virus, inevitably there would be some that did. Vaccines—just beginning their rollout—might be less effective against new variants, and while modern vaccine technology did have the capability to adapt promptly to new mutations, any redesign would take time. The decisive blow vaccination was supposed to deliver to the pandemic would be further delayed. There could still be a third wave, or indeed many waves, if new, more aggressive variants emerged before herd immunity could be established.

LESSONS LEARNED

While it was obviously too early to hold a full post-mortem while the pandemic had not yet run its course, there were already valuable lessons we could learn in case there was ever a next time.

We needed to be better prepared. In early 2019 Canada's highly regarded pandemic alert team—the Global Public Health Intelligence Network, whose job it was to detect outbreaks early and alert the government—had effectively been shuttered. In August 2020 the federal government quietly relaunched the agency, together with a review into how it came to be silenced in the first place.

We needed to act quickly and decisively, or by the time we did react it could already be too late. New Zealand took a "go early, go hard" approach from the start and became a shining example of how the virus could be brought to heel by closing borders early and extinguishing chains of transmission within the country. New Zealand used extensive testing, contact tracing and stringent government-managed quarantine early on, and by the end of the year had contained not only the first wave but also the second. Only twenty-five deaths in total were recorded up to the end of 2020—the lowest per capita death rate in the world.

Part of New Zealand's success was an effective communication strategy. Officials were able to explain the complexity of the crisis to the population in clear and unambiguous language, and this ensured cooperation. If Canada had any communication strategy at all beyond daily press briefings by politicians and medical officers of health, it was not obvious. These briefings, while useful for the media, were data packed, long and tedious, and to the average person provided little in the way of clarity.

Changing behaviour is difficult. Radically altering the way we lived required mass education. Rather than finger wagging from politicians, simple messages that appealed to our better natures were much more likely to persuade us to comply with public health directives. But it was December before we saw the first simple messaging appear on television.

In Canada, as elsewhere, racialized communities bore a disproportionate burden of severe or fatal COVID-19 infections—a trend not completely explained by pre-existing medical conditions.[1] In multicultural Toronto, where racialized groups make up half the population, they experienced 82 per cent of infections and 71 per cent of hospitalizations.

The easy explanation was that poorer socio-economic conditions—an established risk factor for COVID-19—were to blame. It was argued that racialized people often lived in crowded accommodations in low-income neighbourhoods and worked in badly paid front-line jobs, the very roles for which they were lauded as unsung heroes during the pandemic.[2] But in the UK, 94 per cent of doctors who died from COVID-19 were from ethnic minorities—a grim statistic clearly not due to socio-economic factors.

A better explanation was that vitamin D deficiency was to blame. While not the only nutrient needed to prevent complications of viral infections, vitamin D is the only one more likely to be deficient in people with darker skin. A 2011 survey by Statistics Canada found that the prevalence of vitamin D deficiency in Canadians was 37.2 per cent overall, but in non-whites it was 60.7 per cent.[3]

It was surprising to see how reluctant public health officials were to confront this issue. "Recent studies on vitamin D, they raise an eyebrow . . . and it's a good question to ask, but it's premature to start making claims about vitamin D and COVID-19," said Dr. Isaac Bogoch, infectious disease specialist at Toronto General Hospital and a well-respected media commentator.[4] But it is not a hypothesis to suggest that a fully functional immune system depends on vitamin D; it is a known and accepted fact that needs no further proof. Vitamin D is an essential nutrient. All biological systems, including the immune system, will be negatively affected if it is unavailable.[5]

We know that people with darker skin are more likely to be vitamin D deficient compared with their white-skinned colleagues and friends, since the melanin in their skin makes it more difficult for them to make vitamin D from sunshine. Not to alert racialized communities to the implications of vitamin D deficiency during the pandemic was possibly unethical and could be construed as racist. It might be construed as racist. In British Columbia doctors were specifically instructed *not* to recommend vitamin D to their patients outside of approved randomized controlled trials.[6]

COVID-19 AND THE SWISS CHEESE MODEL

The Swiss cheese model, popularized by British cognitive psychologist James Reason in the 1990s, is used to explain how multiple layers of protection work together to improve aviation safety. Recently it has been used to help us see how many different public health measures used together build an effective immune barrier, blocking entry of viruses into tissues.

Imagine a packet of Swiss cheese slices. Each slice represents a single layer of protection. In a perfect world each layer would block the virus from access to a host. But, like Swiss cheese, no single layer is perfect—each one contains random holes through which infection can penetrate. But layer the slices one on top of the other—face masks on top of physical distancing, hand-washing and crowd avoidance—and the holes in one slice are blocked by the next, until near total protection is achieved. "It's not really about any single layer of protection or the order of them, but about the additive success of using multiple layers, or cheese slices," says virologist Ian Mackay of the University of Queensland.[7]

The Swiss cheese model can also help us understand the role of nutrition in protecting against disease. Each slice represents a nutrient—protein, vitamin D, omega-3 fats, vitamin C and so on. No one slice can stop disease. But all nutrients together—one slice on top of another—build a solid wall of defence against chronic illnesses, as well as ensuring the optimal functioning of the immune system.

WE ARE ADAPTABLE; WE ARE RESILIENT

If the health catastrophe of the century has taught us anything, it is how quickly we can adapt in a crisis. Overnight we can change how we educate, how we live, how we interact socially. Could the pandemic be our wake-up call to improve our nutrition?

Scientists are pointing out that nutrition is the key to immune resilience and plays a pivotal role in the development of chronic diseases like obesity, diabetes and cardiovascular disease. In turn these diseases and the nutritional inadequacies that go with them increase the risk of serious or fatal complications from COVID-19.

If the pandemic does nothing more than encourage us to turn our focus to improving and optimizing nutrition, it will not have been entirely in vain. We can do this secure in the knowledge that we can slow the deterioration of immunity with age, prevent the development and progression of chronic illnesses, and prime our immune systems for future battles with novel and resourceful pathogens.

ACKNOWLEDGEMENTS

I owe a debt of gratitude to many friends and colleagues for help during the development of this book. I would especially like to thank Drs. Nadine Bukmuz and Linda Rapson, who were kind enough to read various drafts of the manuscript. I thank them for their many thoughtful comments and discussions—their input has been invaluable. Sincere thanks also to Dr. Ira Bernstein for helpful discussions.

For their encouragement and support, I want to thank Beverley Slopen, my literary agent, and my editor at HarperCollins Canada, Patrick Crean. His advice and constant support, especially during the isolation and uncertainty of the pandemic, were, as ever, vital.

During the last year, there has been an unprecedented flood of new scientific papers on the pandemic, and I am grateful to Alan Shar for ongoing help with research.

Lastly, I would like to thank the production staff at Harper-Collins, who went the extra mile to make sure that this book was edited, designed and printed in record time.

Chapter One: An Ill-Prepared World

1. Implementation of the international health regulations (2005): Report of the review committee on the functioning of the international health regulations (2005) in relation to pandemic (H1N1) 2009. Geneva: World Health Organization; 2011. Available from: https://apps.who.int/gb/ebwha/pdf_files/WHA64/A64_10-en.pdf

2. Abbasi K. The scandals of COVID-19. BMJ. 2020;369:m1434.

3. Mahase E. COVID-19: coronavirus was first described in *The BMJ* in 1965. BMJ. 2020;369:m1547.

4. Mahase E. Coronavirus COVID-19 has killed more people than SARS and MERS combined, despite lower case fatality rate. BMJ. 2020;368:m641.

5. Moni MA, Liò P. Network-based analysis of comorbidities risk during an infection: SARS and HIV case studies. BMC Bioinformatics. 2014;15(1):333.

6. Grabowski DC, Mor V. Nursing home care in crisis in the wake of COVID-19. JAMA. 2020;324(1):23–24.

7. Li R, Pei S, Chen B, et al. Substantial undocumented infection facilitates the rapid dissemination of novel coronavirus (SARS-CoV-2). Science. 2020;368(6490):489–93. Epub 2020 Mar 16.

8. Furukawa NW, Brooks JT, Sobel J. Evidence supporting transmission of severe acute respiratory syndrome coronavirus 2 while presymptomatic or asymptomatic. Emerg Infect Dis. 2020 Jul;26(7):e201595. Available from: https://doi.org/10.3201/eid2607.201595.

9.   Bigelow BF, Tang O, Barshick B, et al. Outcomes of universal COVID-19 test-ing following detection of incident cases in 11 long-term care facilities. JAMA Intern Med. 2020 Jul 14:e203738. doi:10.1001/jamainternmed.2020.3738. Epub ahead of print.

10.   Ing AJ, Cocks C, Green JP. COVID-19: in the footsteps of Ernest Shackle-ton. Thorax. 2020 Aug;75(8):693–94. doi: 10.1136/thoraxjnl-2020-215091. Epub 2020 May 27.

11.   Marineli F, Tsoucalas G, Karamanou M, et al. Mary Mallon (1869–1938) and the history of typhoid fever. Ann Gastroenterol. 2013;26(2):132–34.

12.   History of 1918 flu pandemic [Internet]. Atlanta: Centers for Disease Con-trol and Prevention. Available from: https://www.cdc.gov/flu/pandemic-resources/1918-commemoration/1918-pandemic-history.htm.

13.   Saunders-Hastings PR, Krewski D. Reviewing the history of pandemic influ-enza: understanding patterns of emergence and transmission. Pathogens. 2016 Dec 6;5(4):66.

14.   Vaughan WT. Influenza: an epidemiologic study. Baltimore: American Jour-nal of Hygiene; 1921. p. 241.

15.   Milne I. Stacking the coffins: influenza, war and revolution in Ireland, 1918–19. Manchester (GB): Manchester University Press; 2018.

Chapter Two: The Trouble with Viruses

1.   Pasteur L. The germ theory and its application to medicine and surgery. In Eliot CW, editor. Harvard classics, vol. 38: scientific papers by Harvey, Jenner, Lister, Pasteur. New York: Collier; 1910. p. 366.

2.   Hempelmann E, Krafts K. Bad air, amulets and mosquitoes: 2,000 years of changing perspectives on malaria. Malar J. 2013 Jul 9;12:232.

3.   Morono Y, Ito M, Hoshino T, et al. Aerobic microbial life persists in oxic marine sediment as old as 101.5 million years. Nat Commun. 2020 Jul 28;11(1):3626.

4.   Smith EC, Denison MR. Coronaviruses as DNA wannabes: a new model for the regulation of RNA virus replication fidelity. PLoS Pathog. 2013;9(12):e1003760. doi:10.1371/journal.ppat.1003760. Epub 2013 Dec 5.

5.   Legendre M, Bartoli J, Shmakova L, et al. Thirty-thousand-year-old distant relative of giant icosahedral DNA viruses with a pandoravirus morphology. Proc Natl Acad Sci U S A. 2014 Mar;111(11):4274–79.

6.   Fenollar F, Mediannikov O. Emerging infectious diseases in Africa in the 21st century. New Microbes New Infect. 2018 Sep 21;26:S10–S18.

7. Crawford DH. Viruses: a very short introduction. 2nd ed. Oxford (GB): Oxford University Press; 2018.

8. Koonin EV, Martin W. On the origin of genomes and cells within inorganic compartments. Trends Genet. 2005 Dec;21(12):647–54.

9. Harish A, Abroi A, Gough J, et al. Did viruses evolve as a distinct supergroup from common ancestors of cells? Genome Biol Evol. 2016 Aug 27;8(8): 2474–81.

10. Reche I, D'Orta G, Mladenov N, et al. Deposition rates of viruses and bacteria above the atmospheric boundary layer. ISME J. 2018 Apr;12(4):1154–62.

11. Hammond GW, Raddatz RL, Gelskey DE. Impact of atmospheric dispersion and transport of viral aerosols on the epidemiology of influenza. Rev Infect Dis. 1989 May–Jun;11(3):494–97.

12. Sandler NG, Douek DC. Microbial translocation in HIV infection: causes, consequences and treatment opportunities. Nat Rev Microbiol. 2012 Sep; 10(9):655–56.

13. Huang C, Wang Y, Li X, et al. Clinical features of patients infected with 2019 novel coronavirus in Wuhan, China. Lancet. 2020 Feb 15;395(10223):497–506. Erratum in Lancet. 2020 Feb 15;395(10223):496.

14. Tennant SM, Hartland EL, Phumoonna T, et al. Influence of gastric acid on susceptibility to infection with ingested bacterial pathogens. Infect Immun. 2008;76(2):639–45. doi:10.1128/IAI.01138-07.

15. Wang KN, Bell JS, Tan ECK, et al. Proton pump inhibitors and infection-related hospitalizations among residents of long-term care facilities: a case-control study. Drugs Aging. 2019 Nov;36(11):1027–34.

16. Almario CV, Chey WD, Spiegel BMR. Increased risk of COVID-19 among users of proton pump inhibitors. Am J Gastroenterol. 2020 Oct; 115(10):1707–15.

17. Wageningen University and Research Centre. One virus particle is enough to cause infectious disease. ScienceDaily; 2009. Available from: https://www.sciencedaily.com/releases/2009/03/090313150254.htm.

18. Mok HP, Lever A. Waking up the sleepers: HIV latency and reactivation. J Formos Med Assoc. 2008;107(12):909–14.

19. White DW, Suzanne Beard R, Barton ES. Immune modulation during latent herpesvirus infection. Immunol Rev. 2012;245(1):189–208.

20. Sandalova E, Laccabue D, Boni C, et al. Contribution of herpesvirus specific CD8 T cells to anti-viral T cell response in humans. PLoS Pathog. 2010 Aug 19;6(8):e1001051.

21. White DW, Keppel CR, Schneider SE, et al. Latent herpesvirus infection arms NK cells. Blood. 2010 Jun 3;115(22):4377–83.

22. Traylen CM, Patel HR, Fondaw W, et al. Virus reactivation: a panoramic view in human infections. Future Virol. 2011;6(4):451–63.

23. *Ibid.*

24. Egan KP, Wu S, Wigdahl B, et al. Immunological control of herpes simplex virus infections. J Neurovirol. 2013 Aug;19(4):328–45.

25. Can cold sores be prevented? [Internet]. In: InformedHealth.org. Cologne, Germany: Institute for Quality and Efficiency in Health Care (IQWiG); 2006–. Available from: https://www.ncbi.nlm.nih.gov/books/NBK525765/.

26. Lamey PJ, Biagioni PA. Relationship between iron status and recrudescent herpes labialis. Eur J Clin Microbiol Infect Dis. 1995 Jul;14(7):604–5.

27. Glowacka I, Bertram S, Herzog P, et al. Differential downregulation of ACE2 by the spike proteins of severe acute respiratory syndrome coronavirus and human coronavirus NL63. J Virol. 2010 Jan;84(2):1198–1205.

28. Hambleton S, Steinberg SP, LaRussa PS, et al. Risk of herpes zoster in adults immunized with varicella vaccine. J Infect Dis. 2008 Mar 1;197 Suppl 2:S196–99.

29. Fleming A. On the antibacterial action of cultures of a penicillium, with special reference to their use in the isolation of B. influenzae. Br J Exp Pathol. 1929;10(3):226–36.

30. Lobanovska M, Pilla G. Penicillin's discovery and antibiotic resistance: lessons for the future? Yale J Biol Med. 2017 Mar 29;90(1):135–45.

31. The body's ecosystem [Internet]. The Scientist. 2014 [cited 2020 Apr 20]. Available from: https://www.the-scientist.com/features/the-bodys-ecosystem-37085.

32. Nikoopour E, Singh B. Reciprocity in microbiome and immune system interactions and its implications in disease and health. Inflamm Allergy Drug Targets. 2014 Mar;13(2):94–104.

33. Guinane CM, Cotter PD. Role of the gut microbiota in health and chronic gastrointestinal disease: understanding a hidden metabolic organ. Therap Adv Gastroenterol. 2013 Jul;6(4):295–308.

34. Lee KH, Gordon A, Shedden K, et al. The respiratory microbiome and susceptibility to influenza virus infection. PLoS One. 2019 Jan 9;14(1):e0207898.

35. Palleja A, Mikkelsen KH, Forslund SK, et al. Recovery of gut microbiota of healthy adults following antibiotic exposure. Nat Microbiol. 2018 Nov; 3(11):1255–65.

36. Davies J, Davies D. Origins and evolution of antibiotic resistance. Microbiol Mol Biol Rev. 2010 Sep;74(3):417–33.

37. Qiao M, Ying GG, Singer AC, et al. Review of antibiotic resistance in China and its environment. Environ Int. 2018 Jan;110:160–72.

38. Hoffmann M, Kleine-Weber H, Pöhlmann S. A multibasic cleavage site in the spike protein of SARS-CoV-2 is essential for infection of human lung cells. Mol Cell. 2020 May 21;78(4):779–84.e5.

39. Coutard B, Valle C, de Lamballerie X, et al. The spike glycoprotein of the new coronavirus 2019-nCoV contains a furin-like cleavage site absent in CoV of the same clade. Antiviral Res. 2020 Apr;176:104742.

40. Beigel JH, Tomashek KM, Dodd LE, et al. Remdesivir for the treatment of Covid-19—preliminary report. N Engl J Med. 2020 May 22. doi:10.1056/ NEJMoa2007764.

41. The characteristics of pandemic pathogens. Baltimore: Johns Hopkins Bloomberg School of Public Health; 2018. Available from: https://www .centerforhealthsecurity.org/our-work/pubs_archive/pubs-pdfs/2018/180510 -pandemic-pathogens-report.pdf

42. Adalja AA, Watson M, Toner ES, et al. Characteristics of microbes most likely to cause pandemics and global catastrophes. Curr Top Microbiol Immunol. 2019;424:1–20.

Chapter Three: The Immune System Fights Back

1. Nicholson LB. The immune system. Essays Biochem. 2016 Oct 31;60(3): 275–301.

2. O'Neill LA, Golenbock D, Bowie AG. The history of Toll-like receptors— redefining innate immunity. Nat Rev Immunol. 2013 Jun;13(6): 453–60.

3. Christmas P. Toll-like receptors: sensors that detect infection. Nature Education. 2010;3(9):85.

4. Gaudino SJ, Kumar P. Cross-talk between antigen presenting cells and T cells impacts intestinal homeostasis, bacterial infections, and tumorigenesis. Front Immunol. 2019 Mar 6;10:360.

5.   Gibbons DL, Haque SF, Silberzahn T, et al. Neonates harbour highly active gammadelta T cells with selective impairments in preterm infants. Eur J Immunol. 2009 Jul;39(7):1794–1806.

6.   Bahadoran A, Lee SH, Wang SM, et al. Immune responses to influenza virus and its correlation to age and inherited factors. Front Microbiol. 2016 Nov 22;7:1841.

7.   Suzuki S, Eastwood GM, Bailey M, et al. Paracetamol therapy and outcome of critically ill patients: a multicenter retrospective observational study. Crit Care. 2015 Apr 13;19(1):162.

8.   Bohmwald K, Gálvez NMS, Canedo-Marroquín G, et al. Contribution of cytokines to tissue damage during human respiratory syncytial virus infection. Front Immunol. 2019 Mar 18;10:452.

9.   Stephen-Victor E, Das M, Karnam A, et al. Potential of regulatory T-cell-based therapies in the management of severe COVID-19. Eur Respir J. 2020 Sep 3;56(3):2002182.

10. Wing K, Sakaguchi S. Regulatory T cells exert checks and balances on self tolerance and autoimmunity. Nat Immunol. 2010 Jan;11(1):7–13.

11. Smatti MK, Cyprian FS, Nasrallah GK, et al. Viruses and autoimmunity: a review on the potential interaction and molecular mechanisms. Viruses. 2019 Aug 19;11(8):762.

12. Riedel S. Edward Jenner and the history of smallpox and vaccination. Proc (Bayl Univ Med Cent). 2005 Jan;18(1):21–25. doi:10.1080/08998280 .2005.11928028.

13. Gross CP, Sepkowitz KA. The myth of the medical breakthrough: smallpox, vaccination, and Jenner reconsidered. Int J Infect Dis. 1998 Jul–Sep;3(1):54–60.

14. Greenwood B. The contribution of vaccination to global health: past, present and future. Philos Trans R Soc Lond B Biol Sci. 2014 May 12; 369(1645):20130433.

15. Jung F, Krieger V, Hufert FT, et al. Herd immunity or suppression strategy to combat COVID-19. Clin Hemorheol Microcirc. 2020;75(1):13–17.

16. Coronavirus: Sweden's Tegnell admits too many died [Internet]. BBC News. BBC; 2020. Available from: https://www.bbc.com/news/world-europe-52903717.

17. WHO coronavirus disease (COVID-19) dashboard [Internet]. World Health Organization; 2020. Available from: https://covid19.who.int/?gclid=EAIaI QobChMIqKLOtJae7QIVhIXICh3IagDWEAAYASAAEgL2XfD_BwE.

18. Bruggeman L, Cathey L. Former Stanford colleagues warn Dr. Scott Atlas fosters "falsehoods and misrepresentations of science." ABC News. ABC News Network; 2020. Available from: https://abcnews.go.com/Politics/stanford-colleagues-warn-dr-scott-atlas-fosters-falsehoods/story?id=72926212.

19. Phan T. Genetic diversity and evolution of SARS-CoV-2. Infect Genet Evol. 2020 Jul;81:104260.

20. Montelongo-Jauregui D, Vila T, Sultan AS, et al. Convalescent serum therapy for COVID-19: a 19th century remedy for a 21st century disease. PLoS Pathog. 2020 Aug 12;16(8):e1008735.

21. *Ibid.*

22. Pathak EB. Convalescent plasma is ineffective for covid-19. BMJ. 2020 Oct 22;371:m4072

23. Clinical trials of monoclonal antibodies to prevent COVID-19 now enrolling [Internet]. National Institutes of Health. US Department of Health and Human Services; 2020 Aug 10. Available from: https://www.nih.gov/news-events/news-releases/clinical-trials-monoclonal-antibodies-prevent-covid-19-now-enrolling.

24. Marik PE. Steroids for sepsis: yes, no or maybe. J Thorac Dis. 2018 Apr;10 (Suppl 9):S1070–S1073. doi: 10.21037/jtd.2018.04.35.

25. Dexamethasone for COVID-19: preliminary findings. Drug Ther Bull. 2020 Sep;58(9):133.

26. Blanco-Melo D, Nilsson-Payant BE, Liu WC, et al. Imbalanced host response to SARS-CoV-2 drives development of COVID-19. Cell. 2020 May 28; 181(5):1036–45.e9.

27. Meng Z, Wang T, Li C, et al. An experimental trial of recombinant human interferon alpha nasal drops to prevent coronavirus disease 2019 in medical staff in an epidemic area. [Preprint]. Available from: https://www.medrxiv.org/content/10.1101/2020.04.11.20061473v2.

28. Single-blind study of a single dose of peginterferon lambda-1a compared with placebo in outpatients with mild COVID-19 (COVID-lambda)—full text view—ClinicalTrials.gov. Stanford University; 2020. Available from: https://clinicaltrials.gov/ct2/show/NCT04331899?term=stanford+lambda.

29. Wadman M. Can boosting interferons, the body's frontline virus fighters, beat COVID-19? [Internet]. Science. 2020. Available from: https://www.sciencemag.org/news/2020/07/can-boosting-interferons-body-s-frontline-virus-fighters-beat-covid-19.

30. Broggi A, Ghosh S, Sposito B, et al. Type III interferons disrupt the lung epithelial barrier upon viral recognition. Science. 2020 Aug 7;369(6504): 706–12.

31. Keller MJ, Kitsis EA, Arora S, et al. Effect of systemic glucocorticoids on mortality or mechanical ventilation in patients with COVID-19. J Hosp Med. 2020 Aug;15(8);489–93.

32. Hodgson J. The pandemic pipeline. Nat Biotechnol. 2020 May;38(5):523–32.

33. Folegatti PM, Ewer KJ, Aley PK, et al. Oxford COVID Vaccine Trial Group. Safety and immunogenicity of the ChAdOx1 nCoV-19 vaccine against SARS-CoV-2: a preliminary report of a phase 1/2, single-blind, randomised controlled trial. Lancet. 2020 Aug 15;396(10249):467–78.

34. Mehndiratta MM, Mehndiratta P, Pande R. Poliomyelitis: historical facts, epidemiology, and current challenges in eradication. Neurohospitalist. 2014 Oct;4(4):223–29.

35. Poliomyelitis. In: Hamborsky J, Kroger A, Wolfe C, editors. Epidemiology and prevention of vaccine-preventable diseases. 13th ed. Washington (DC): US Department of Health & Human Services, Centers for Disease Control and Prevention; 2015. p. 297–310. Available from: https://www.cdc.gov/vaccines/pubs/pinkbook/downloads/polio.pdf.

36. Post-polio syndrome [Internet]. Mayo Clinic. Mayo Foundation for Medical Education and Research; 2020. Available from: https://www.mayoclinic.org/diseases-conditions/post-polio-syndrome/symptoms-causes/syc-20355669.

37. Post-polio syndrome fact sheet [Internet]. Bethesda (MD): National Institute of Neurological Disorders and Stroke. US Department of Health & Human Services; 2012. Available from: https://www.ninds.nih.gov/Disorders/Patient-Caregiver-Education/Fact-Sheets/Post-Polio-Syndrome-Fact-Sheet.

38. Moldofsky H, Patcai J. Chronic widespread musculoskeletal pain, fatigue, depression and disordered sleep in chronic post-SARS syndrome; a case-controlled study. BMC Neurol. 2011 Mar 24;11:37.

Chapter Four: Medicine and the Lost Art of Nutrition

1. Prevalence of chronic diseases among Canadian adults [Internet]. Public Health Agency of Canada. Government of Canada; 2019. Available from: https://www.canada.ca/en/public-health/services/chronic-diseases/prevalence-canadian-adults-infographic-2019.html.

2. Sze S, Pellicori P, Zhang J, et al. The impact of malnutrition on short-term morbidity and mortality in ambulatory patients with heart failure. Am J Clin Nutr. 2020 Nov 24:nqaa311.

3. Katona P, Katona-Apte J. The interaction between nutrition and infection. Clin Infect Dis. 2008 May 15;46(10):1582–88.

4. Allard, JP, Keller H, Jeejeebhoy KN, et al. Malnutrition at hospital admission-contributors and effect on length of stay: a prospective cohort study from the Canadian Malnutrition Task Force. JPEN J Parenter Enteral Nutr. 2016 May;40(4):487–97.

5. Bencivenga L, Rengo G, Varricchi G. Elderly at time of COronaVIrus disease 2019 (COVID-19): possible role of immunosenescence and malnutrition. Geroscience. 2020 Aug;42(4):1089–92.

6. Keller HH. Malnutrition in institutionalized elderly: how and why? J Am Geriatr Soc. 1993 Nov;41(11):1212–18.

7. Leij-Halfwerk S, Verwijs MH, van Houdt S, et al. Prevalence of protein-energy malnutrition risk in European older adults in community, residential and hospital settings, according to 22 malnutrition screening tools validated for use in adults ≥65 years: a systematic review and meta-analysis. Maturitas. 2019 Aug;126:80–89.

8. Damião R, Santos ÁDS, Matijasevich A, et al. Factors associated with risk of malnutrition in the elderly in south-eastern Brazil. Rev Bras Epidemiol. 2017 Oct–Dec;20(4):598–610.

9. Chandra RK. Nutrition and the immune system: an introduction. Am J Clin Nutr. 1997 Aug;66(2):460S-463S.

10. Zhou F, Yu T, Du R, et al. Clinical course and risk factors for mortality of adult inpatients with COVID-19 in Wuhan, China: a retrospective cohort study. Lancet. 2020 Mar 28;395 (10229):1054–62.

11. Malhotra A, Redberg RF, Meier P. Saturated fat does not clog the arteries: coronary heart disease is a chronic inflammatory condition, the risk of which can be effectively reduced from healthy lifestyle interventions. Br J Sports Med. 2017 Aug;51(15):1111–12.

12. Geiker NRW, Larsen ML, Dyerberg J, et al. Egg consumption, cardiovascular diseases and type 2 diabetes. Eur J Clin Nutr. 2018 Jan;72(1):44–56.

13. Shih CW, Hauser ME, Aronica L, et al. Changes in blood lipid concentrations associated with changes in intake of dietary saturated fat in the context

of a healthy low-carbohydrate weight-loss diet: a secondary analysis of the Diet Intervention Examining The Factors Interacting with Treatment Success (DIETFITS) trial. Am J Clin Nutr. 2019 Feb 1;109(2):433–41.

14. Otto MCDO, Lemaitre RN, Song X, et al. Serial measures of circulating bio-markers of dairy fat and total and cause-specific mortality in older adults: the Cardiovascular Health Study. Am J Clin Nutr. 2018 Sep 11;108(3):476–84.

15. Jastrzebski Z, Kortas J, Kaczor K, Antosiewicz J. Vitamin D supplementation causes a decrease in blood cholesterol in professional rowers. J Nutr Sci Vita-minol (Tokyo). 2016;62(2):88–92.

16. Volek JS, Sharman MJ, Gómez AL, et al. An isoenergetic very low carbohy-drate diet improves serum HDL cholesterol and triacylglycerol concentra-tions, the total cholesterol to HDL cholesterol ratio and postprandial pipemic responses compared with a low fat diet in normal weight, normolipidemic women. J Nutr. 2003 Sep;133(9):2756–61.

17. Gjuladin-Hellon T, Davies IG, Penson P, et al. Effects of carbohydrate-restricted diets on low-density lipoprotein cholesterol levels in overweight and obese adults: a systematic review and meta-analysis. Nutr Rev. 2019 Mar 1; 77(3):161–80.

18. Diet, nutrition and the prevention of chronic diseases: report of a joint WHO/FAO expert consultation. Geneva: World Health Organization; 2003. WHO Technical Report Series, No. 916 (TRS 916). Available from: https://www.who.int/dietphysicalactivity/publications/trs916/summary/en/.

19. Vetter ML, Herring SJ, Sood M, et al. What do resident physicians know about nutrition? An evaluation of attitudes, self-perceived proficiency and knowledge. J Am Coll Nutr. 2008 Apr;27(2):287–98. doi:10.1080/07315724.2008.10719702.

20. Adams KM, Kohlmeier M, Zeisel SH. Nutrition education in U.S. medical schools: latest update of a national survey. Acad Med. 2010 Sep;85(9):1537–42.

21. Gramlich LM, Olstad DL, Nasser R, et al. Medical students' perceptions of nutrition education in Canadian universities. Appl Physiol Nutr Metab. 2010 Jun;35(3):336–43.

22. Broad J, Wallace M. Nutrition and public health in medical education in the UK: reflections and next steps. Public Health Nutr. 2018 Sep;21(13):2523–25.

23. Orimo H, Ueno T, Yoshida H, et al. Nutrition education in Japanese medical schools: a follow-up survey. Asia Pac J Clin Nutr. 2013;22(1):144–49.

24. Blunt SB, Kafatos A. Clinical nutrition education of doctors and medical students: solving the catch 22. Adv Nutr. 2019 Mar 1;10(2):345–50.

25. McCarrison R. Nutrition in health and disease. Br Med J. 1936 Sep 26; 2(3951):611–15.

26. McCarrison R. Studies in deficiency disease. London: Henry Frowde and Hodder & Stoughton; 1921.

27. Crowley J, Ball L, Hiddink GJ. Nutrition in medical education: a systematic review. Lancet Planet Health. 2019 Sep;3(9):e379–e389.

28. Israels LG, Israels ED. Apoptosis. Stem Cells. 1999;17(5):306–13.

29. Williams JM, Duckworth CA, Burkitt MD, et al. Epithelial cell shedding and barrier function: a matter of life and death at the small intestinal villus tip. Vet Pathol. 2015 May;52(3):445–55.

30. Rosales C. Neutrophil: a cell with many roles in inflammation or several cell types? Front Physiol. 2018 Feb 20;9:113.

31. Ginter E, Simko V. New data on harmful effects of trans-fatty acids. Bratisl Lek Listy. 2016;117(5):251–53.

32. Chen CL, Tetri LH, Neuschwander-Tetri BA, et al. A mechanism by which dietary trans fats cause atherosclerosis. J Nutr Biochem. 2011 Jul;22(7):649–55.

33. MacKay D, Miller AL. Nutritional support for wound healing. Altern Med Rev. 2003 Nov;8(4):359–77.

34. Wurtman RJ, Hefti F, Melamed E. Precursor control of neurotransmitter synthesis. Pharmacol Rev. 1980 Dec;32(4):315–35.

35. Demelash S. The role of micronutrient for depressed patients. J Neuropsychopharmacol Mental Health. 2017;2(1):116.

36. Młyniec K, Davies CL, de Agüero Sánchez IG, et al. Essential elements in depression and anxiety. Part I. Pharmacol Rep. 2014 Aug;66(4):534–44.

37. Saran S, Gupta BS, Philip R, et al. Effect of hypothyroidism on female reproductive hormones. Indian J Endocrinol Metab. 2016 Jan–Feb; 20(1): 108–13.

38. Pałkowska-Goździk E, Lachowicz K, Rosołowska-Huszcz D. Effects of dietary protein on thyroid axis activity. Nutrients. 2017 Dec 22;10(1):5.

39. Trotti LM. Restless legs syndrome and sleep-related movement disorders. Continuum (Minneap Minn). 2017 Aug;23(4, Sleep Neurology):1005–16.

40. Burman D. Sleep disorders: restless legs syndrome. FP Essent. 2017 Sep;460:29–32.

41.   He Q, Chen X, Wu T, et al. Risk of dementia in long-term benzodiazepine users: evidence from a meta-analysis of observational studies. J Clin Neurol. 2019 Jan;15(1):9–19.

42.   Lehvilä P. Bruxism and magnesium. Literature review and case reports. Proc Finn Dent Soc. 1974 Dec;70(6):217–24.

43.   Cavalcante AL, Siqueira RM, Araujo JC, et al. Role of NMDA receptors in the trigeminal pathway, and the modulatory effect of magnesium in a model of rat temporomandibular joint arthritis. Eur J Oral Sci. 2013 Nov 30;121(6):573–83.

44.   Sinniah D. Magnesium deficiency: a possible cause of restless leg syndrome in haemodialysis patients. Intern Med J. 2015 Apr;45(4):467–68.

45.   Rude RK. Magnesium metabolism and deficiency. Endocrinol Metab Clin North Am. 1993 Jun;22(2):377–95.

46.   DiNicolantonio JJ, O'Keefe JH, Wilson W. Subclinical magnesium deficiency: a principal driver of cardiovascular disease and a public health crisis. Open Heart. 2018 Jan 13;5(1):e000668.

47.   Workinger JL, Doyle RP, Bortz J. Challenges in the diagnosis of magnesium status. Nutrients. 2018 Sep 1;10(9):1202.

48.   Senate Document 264, 74th Cong., 2nd Sess. (1936) [cited 2020 Oct 7]. Available from: https://www.prismnet.com/~lenb/centurynutrition/senate 264.htm.

49.   Martínez Steele E, Popkin BM, Swinburn B, et al. The share of ultra-processed foods and the overall nutritional quality of diets in the US: evidence from a nationally representative cross-sectional study. Popul Health Metr. 2017 Feb 14;15(1):6.

50.   Gröber U. Magnesium and drugs. Int J Mol Sci. 2019 Apr 28;20(9):2094.

51.   Cuciureanu MD, Vink R. Magnesium and stress. In: Vink R, Nechifor M, editors. Magnesium in the central nervous system [Internet]. Adelaide: University of Adelaide Press; 2011. Available from: https://www.ncbi.nlm.nih.gov/books/NBK507250.

52.   Seelig MS. Consequences of magnesium deficiency on the enhancement of stress reactions; preventive and therapeutic implications (a review). J Am Coll Nutr. 1994 Oct;13(5):429–46.

53.   Pickering G, Mazur A, Trousselard M, et al. Magnesium status and stress: the vicious circle concept revisited. Nutrients. 2020 Nov 28;12(12):3672.

54.   Blumberg J, Heaney RP, Huncharek M, et al. Evidence-based criteria in the nutritional context. Nutr Rev. 2010 Aug;68(8):478–84.

55. Al Alawi AM, Majoni SW, Falhammar H. Magnesium and human health: perspectives and research directions. Int J Endocrinol. 2018 Apr 16; 2018:9041694.

56. Houston M. The role of magnesium in hypertension and cardiovascular disease. J Clin Hypertens (Greenwich). 2011 Nov;13(11):843–47.

57. Rosanoff A, Plesset MR. Oral magnesium supplements decrease high blood pressure (SBP>155 mmHg) in hypertensive subjects on anti-hypertensive medications: a targeted meta-analysis. Magnes Res. 2013 Jul–Sep;26(3):93–99.

58. Viering DHHM, de Baaij JHF, Walsh SB, et al. Genetic causes of hypomagnesemia, a clinical overview. Pediatr Nephrol. 2017 Jul;32(7):1123–35.

59. Gröber U. Magnesium and drugs. Int J Mol Sci. 2019 Apr 28;20(9):2094.

60. Seelig MS. Consequences of magnesium deficiency on the enhancement of stress reactions; preventive and therapeutic implications (a review). J Am Coll Nutr. 1994 Oct;13(5):429–46.

61. Ordovas JM, Ferguson LR, Tai ES, et al. Personalised nutrition and health. BMJ. 2018 Jun 13;361:bmj.k2173.

62. Workinger JL, Doyle RP, Bortz J. Challenges in the diagnosis of magnesium status. Nutrients. 2018 Sep 1;10(9):1202.

63. *Ibid.*

64. Singh RB. Effect of dietary magnesium supplementation in the prevention of coronary heart disease and sudden cardiac death. Magnes Trace Elem. 1990;9(3):143–51.

65. Efstratiadis G, Sarigianni M, Gougourelas I. Hypomagnesemia and cardiovascular system. Hippokratia. 2006 Oct;10(4):147–52.

66. Briggs RD, Rubenberg ML, O'Neal RM, et al. Myocardial infarction in patients treated with Sippy and other high-milk diets: an autopsy study of fifteen hospitals in the U.S.A. and Great Britain. Circulation. 1960 Apr;21:538–42.

67. Saver JL, Kalafut M. Combination therapies and the theoretical limits of evidence-based medicine. Neuroepidemiology. 2001 May;20(2):57–64.

68. Cashman JD. Diet, nutrition, and bone health. J. Nutr. 2007 Nov;137 (11 Suppl): 2507S–12S.

69. Hébert JR, Frongillo EA, Adams SA, et al. Perspective: randomized controlled trials are not a panacea for diet-related research. Adv Nutr. 2016 May 16;7(3):423–32.

70. Allan GM, Cranston L, Lindblad A, et al. Vitamin D: a narrative review examining the evidence for ten beliefs. J Gen Intern Med. 2016 Jul;31(7):780–91.

71.   Neitz R. Vitamin D may not be the great solution to health problems [Internet]. Edmonton: University of Alberta. Faculty of Medicine & Dentistry; 2016. Available from: https://www.ualberta.ca/medicine/news/2016/june/vitamin-d-may-not-be-the-great-solution-to-health-problems.html.

72.   Prietl B, Treiber G, Pieber TR, et al. Vitamin D and immune function. Nutrients. 2013 Jul 5;5(7):2502–21.

73.   Harmon K. Another reason vitamin D is important: it gets T cells going [Internet]. Scientific American. 2010. Available from: https://blogs.scientificamerican.com/observations/another-reason-vitamin-d-is-important-it-gets-t-cells-going/.

74.   Maggini S, Pierre A, Calder PC. Immune function and micronutrient requirements change over the life course. Nutrients. 2018 Oct 17;10(10):1531.

75.   Richardson DP, Lovegrove JA. Nutritional status of micronutrients as a possible and modifiable risk factor for COVID-19: a UK perspective. Br J Nutr. 2020 Aug 20:1–7.

Chapter Five: Good Food; Healing Food

1.   Maggini S, Pierre A, Calder PC. Immune function and micronutrient requirements change over the life course. Nutrients. 2018 Oct 17;10(10):1531.

2.   Pawelec G. Age and immunity: What is "immunosenescence"? Exp Gerontol. 2018 May;105:4–9.

3.   Maijó M, Clements SJ, Ivory K, et al. Nutrition, diet and immunosenescence. Mech Ageing Dev. 2014 Mar–Apr;136–37:116–28.

4.   Livshits G, Kalinkovich A. Inflammaging as a common ground for the development and maintenance of sarcopenia, obesity, cardiomyopathy and dysbiosis. Ageing Res Rev. 2019 Dec;56:100980.

5.   GBD 2017 Diet Collaborators. Health effects of dietary risks in 195 countries, 1990–2017: a systematic analysis for the Global Burden of Disease Study 2017. Lancet. 2019 May 11;393(10184):1958–72.

6.   McMacken M. Food as medicine: nutrition to prevent and reverse chronic disease. Paper presented at: ACP Internal Medicine Annual Meeting; 2018 April 19–21; New Orleans.

7.   Calder PC, Bosco N, Bourdet-Sicard R, et al. Health relevance of the modification of low grade inflammation in ageing (inflammageing) and the role of nutrition. Ageing Res Rev. 2017 Nov;40:95–119.

8. Fries E, Green P, Bowen DJ. What did I eat yesterday? Determinants of accuracy in 24-hour food memories. Applied Cognitive Psychology. 1995 Apr:9(2):143–55.

9. Jacobs DR Jr, Steffen LM. Nutrients, foods, and dietary patterns as exposures in research: a framework for food synergy. Am J Clin Nutr. 2003 Sep;78(3 Suppl):508S–13S.

10. Ng M, Fleming T, Robinson M, et al. Global, regional, and national prevalence of overweight and obesity in children and adults during 1980–2013: a systematic analysis for the Global Burden of Disease Study 2013. Lancet. 2014 Aug 30;384(9945):766–81.

11. Sturm R. The effects of obesity, smoking, and drinking on medical problems and costs. Health Aff (Millwood). 2002 Mar–Apr;21(2):245–53.

12. Mathis D. Immunological goings-on in visceral adipose tissue. Cell Metab. 2013 Jun 4;17(6):851–59.

13. Saltiel AR, Olefsky JM. Inflammatory mechanisms linking obesity and metabolic disease. J Clin Invest. 2017 Jan 3;127(1):1–4.

14. De Lorenzo A, Del Gobbo V, Premrov MG, et al. Normal-weight obese syndrome: early inflammation? Am J Clin Nutr. 2007 Jan;85(1):40–45.

15. Rosen GM, Pou S, Ramos CL, et al. Free radicals and phagocytic cells. FASEB J. 1995 Feb;9(2):200–209.

16. Dunnill C, Patton T, Brennan J, et al. Reactive oxygen species (ROS) and wound healing: the functional role of ROS and emerging ROS-modulating technologies for augmentation of the healing process. Int Wound J. 2017 Feb;14(1):89–96.

17. Lopez-Jimenez F. Can coenzyme Q10 prevent statin side effects? [Internet]. Mayo Clinic. Mayo Foundation for Medical Education and Research; 2020. Available from: https://www.mayoclinic.org/diseases-conditions/high-blood-cholesterol/expert-answers/coenzyme-q10/faq-20058176.

18. Calder PC. Nutrition, immunity and COVID-19. BMJ Nutr Prev Health. 2020 May 20;3(1):74–92.

19. Tosti V, Bertozzi B, Fontana L. Health benefits of the Mediterranean diet: metabolic and molecular mechanisms. J Gerontol A Biol Sci Med Sci. 2018 Mar 2;73(3):318–26.

20. Calder PC. Nutrition, immunity and COVID-19. BMJ Nutr Prev Health. 2020 May 20;3(1):74–92.

21. Oyebode O, Gordon-Dseagu V, Walker A, et al. Fruit and vegetable consumption and all-cause, cancer and CVD mortality: analysis of Health Survey for England data. J Epidemiol Community Health. 2014 Sep;68(9):856–62.

22. Food guide snapshot [Internet]. Canada's food guide. Health Canada; 2020. Available from: https://food-guide.canada.ca/en/food-guide-snapshot/.

23. Martucci M, Ostan R, Biondi F, et al. Mediterranean diet and inflammaging within the hormesis paradigm. Nutr Rev. 2017 Jun 1;75(6):442–55.

24. Brown MJ, Ferruzzi MG, Nguyen ML, et al. Carotenoid bioavailability is higher from salads ingested with full-fat than with fat-reduced salad dressings as measured with electrochemical detection. Am J Clin Nutr. 2004 Aug;80(2):396–403.

25. Bodey B, Bodey B Jr, Siegel SE, Kaiser HE. Involution of the mammalian thymus, one of the leading regulators of aging. In Vivo. 1997 Sep-Oct;11(5):421-40

26. Dong X, Milholland B, Vijg J. Evidence for a limit to human lifespan. Nature. 2016 Oct 13;538(7624):257–59.

27. Nunes-Alves C, Nobrega C, Behar SM, et al. Tolerance has its limits: how the thymus copes with infection. Trends Immunol. 2013 Oct;34(10):502–10.

28. Velardi E, Tsai JJ, van den Brink MRM. T cell regeneration after immunological injury. Nat Rev Immunol. 2020 Oct 23:1–15.

29. Cunningham-Rundles S, McNeeley DF, Moon A. Mechanisms of nutrient modulation of the immune response. J Allergy Clin Immunol. 2005 Jun; 115(6):1119–28.

30. Savino W, Dardenne M. Nutritional imbalances and infections affect the thymus: consequences on T-cell-mediated immune responses. Proc Nutr Soc. 2010 Nov;69(4):636–43.

31. Ganapathy A, Nieves JW. Nutrition and sarcopenia—What do we know? Nutrients. 2020 Jun 11;12(6):1755.

32. Rodriguez NR. Introduction to Protein Summit 2.0: continued exploration of the impact of high-quality protein on optimal health. Am J Clin Nutr. 2015 Jun;101(6):1317S–1319S.

33. Ludwig DS, Dickinson SL, Henschel B, et al. Do lower-carbohydrate diets increase total energy expenditure? An updated and reanalyzed meta-analysis of 29 controlled-feeding studies. J Nutr. 2020 Dec 3:nxaa350.

34. Layman DK, Boileau RA, Erickson DJ, et al. A reduced ratio of dietary carbohydrate to protein improves body composition and blood lipid profiles during weight loss in adult women. J Nutr. 2003 Feb;133(2):411–17.

35. Hurt RT, McClave SA, Martindale RG, et al. Summary points and consensus recommendations from the International Protein Summit. Nutr Clin Pract. 2017 Apr;32(1_suppl):142S–51S.

36. Mazzulla M, Sawan SA, Williamson E, et al. Protein intake to maximize whole-body anabolism during postexercise recovery in resistance-trained men with high habitual intakes is severalfold greater than the current recommended dietary allowance. J Nutr. 2020 Mar 1;150(3):505–11.

37. Mamerow MM, Mettler JA, English KL, et al. Dietary protein distribution positively influences 24-h muscle protein synthesis in healthy adults. J Nutr. 2014 Jun;144(6):876–80.

38. White RR, Hall MB. Nutritional and greenhouse gas impacts of removing animals from US agriculture. Proc Natl Acad Sci USA. 2017 Nov 28; 114(48):E10301–8.

39. Mozaffarian D, Rimm EB, Herrington DM. Dietary fats, carbohydrate, and progression of coronary atherosclerosis in postmenopausal women. Am J Clin Nutr. 2004 Nov;80(5):1175–84.

40. Malhotra A, Redberg RF, Meier P. Saturated fat does not clog the arteries: coronary heart disease is a chronic inflammatory condition, the risk of which can be effectively reduced from healthy lifestyle interventions. Br J Sports Med. 2017 Aug;51(15):1111–12.

41. Wilkinson SB, Tarnopolsky MA, Macdonald MJ, et al. Consumption of fluid skim milk promotes greater muscle protein accretion after resistance exercise than does consumption of an isonitrogenous and isoenergetic soy-protein beverage. Am J Clin Nutr. 2007 Apr;85(4):1031–40.

42. Jafar N, Edriss H, Nugent K. The effect of short-term hyperglycemia on the innate immune system. Am J Med Sci. 2016 Feb;351(2):201–11.

43. Lennerz BS, Koutnik AP, Azova S, et al. Carbohydrate restriction for diabetes: rediscovering centuries-old wisdom. J Clin Invest. 2021 Jan 4;131(1):e142246.

44. Zafar MI, Mills KE, Zheng J, et al. Low-glycemic index diets as an intervention for diabetes: a systematic review and meta-analysis. Am J Clin Nutr. 2019 Oct 1;110(4):891–902.

45. Unwin D, Khalid AA, Unwin J, et al. Insights from a general practice service evaluation supporting a lower carbohydrate diet in patients with type 2 diabetes mellitus and prediabetes: a secondary analysis of routine clinic data including HbA1c, weight and prescribing over 6 years. BMJ Nutr Prev Health. 2020 Nov 2:bmjnph-2020-000072.

46. Grotto D, Zied E. The Standard American Diet and its relationship to the health status of Americans. Nutr Clin Pract. 2010 Dec;25(6):603–12.

47. Marriott BP, Olsho L, Hadden L, et al. Intake of added sugars and selected nutrients in the United States, National Health and Nutrition Examination Survey (NHANES) 2003–2006. Crit Rev Food Sci Nutr. 2010 Mar;50(3):228–58.

48. Hawkes C. Uneven dietary development: linking the policies and processes of globalization with the nutrition transition, obesity and diet-related chronic diseases. Global Health. 2006 Mar 28;2:4

49. Li Y, Schoufour J, Wang DD, et al. Healthy lifestyle and life expectancy free of cancer, cardiovascular disease, and type 2 diabetes: prospective cohort study. BMJ. 2020 Jan 8;368:l6669.

Chapter Six: Nutritional Supplements and Immunity

1. Korber B, Fischer WM, Gnanakaran S, et al. Spike mutation pipeline reveals the emergence of a more transmissible form of SARS-CoV-2. bioRxiv 2020.04.29.069054 [Preprint]. 2020.

2. Long SW, Olsen RJ, Christensen PA, et al. Molecular architecture of early dissemination and massive second wave of the SARS-CoV-2 virus in a major metropolitan area. medRxiv 2020.09.22.20199125 [Preprint]. 2020.

3. Thieme CJ, Anft M, Paniskaki K, et al. Robust T cell response toward spike, membrane, and nucleocapsid SARS-CoV-2 proteins is not associated with recovery in critical COVID-19 patients. Cell Rep Med. 2020 Sep 22;1(6):100092.

4. Cohen J, Kupferschmidt K. The "very, very bad look" of Remdesivir, the first FDA-approved COVID-19 drug [Internet]. 2020. Available from: https://www.sciencemag.org/news/2020/10/very-very-bad-look-remdesivir-first-fda-approved-covid-19-drug.

5. Coronavirus disease (COVID-19): dexamethasone. Geneva: World Health Organization; 2020. Available from: https://www.who.int/emergencies/diseases/novel-coronavirus-2019/question-and-answers-hub/q-a-detail/coronavirus-disease-covid-19-dexamethasone.

6. Gombart AF, Pierre A, Maggini S. A review of micronutrients and the immune system—working in harmony to reduce the risk of infection. Nutrients. 2020 Jan 16;12(1):236.

7. Richardson DP, Lovegrove JA. Nutritional status of micronutrients as a possible and modifiable risk factor for COVID-19: a UK perspective. Br J Nutr. 2020 Aug 20:1–7.

8. Mora JR, Iwata M, von Andrian UH. Vitamin effects on the immune system: vitamins A and D take centre stage. Nat Rev Immunol. 2008 Sep;8(9):685–98.

9. Maggini S, Pierre A, Calder PC. Immune function and micronutrient requirements change over the life course. Nutrients. 2018 Oct 17;10(10):1531.

10. Zabetakis I, Lordan R, Norton C, et al. COVID-19: The inflammation link and the role of nutrition in potential mitigation. Nutrients. 2020 May 19;12(5):1466.

11. Mikkelsen K, Apostolopoulos V. B vitamins and ageing. Subcell Biochem. 2018;90:451–70.

12. Thomas-Valdés S, Tostes MDGV, Anunciação PC, et al. Association between vitamin deficiency and metabolic disorders related to obesity. Crit Rev Food Sci Nutr. 2017 Oct 13;57(15):3332–43.

13. Bruins MJ, Van Dael P, Eggersdorfer M. The role of nutrients in reducing the risk for noncommunicable diseases during aging. Nutrients. 2019 Jan 4;11(1):85.

14. Fiorino S, Gallo C, Zippi M, et al. Cytokine storm in aged people with CoV-2: possible role of vitamins as therapy or preventive strategy. Aging Clin Exp Res. 2020 Oct;32(10):2115–31.

15. Prevalence of chronic diseases among Canadian adults [Internet]. Public Health Agency of Canada. Government of Canada; 2019. Available from: https://www.canada.ca/en/public-health/services/chronic-diseases/prevalence-canadian-adults-infographic-2019.html.

16. Murphy SP, Yates AA, Atkinson SA, et al. History of nutrition: the long road leading to the dietary reference intakes for the United States and Canada. Adv Nutr. 2016 Jan;7(1):157–68.

17. Institute of Medicine (US) Food and Nutrition Board. How should the recommended dietary allowances be revised? Washington (DC): National Academies Press (US); 1994. Chapter 2, Concepts underlying the recommended dietary allowances. Available from: https://www.ncbi.nlm.nih.gov/books/NBK231420/.

18. Wu D, Lewis ED, Pae M, et al. Nutritional modulation of immune function: analysis of evidence, mechanisms, and clinical relevance. Front Immunol. 2019 Jan 15;9:3160.

19. MacFarlane AJ, Cogswell ME, de Jesus JM, et al. A report of activities related to the dietary reference intakes from the Joint Canada-US Dietary Reference Intakes Working Group. Am J Clin Nutr. 2019 Feb 1;109(2):251–59.

20. Expansion of the dietary reference intake model [Internet]. Washington (DC): National Academies of Sciences; (n.d.). Available from: https://www.nap.edu/resource/25353/interactive/.

21. Kostov K, Halacheva L. Role of magnesium deficiency in promoting atherosclerosis, endothelial dysfunction, and arterial stiffening as risk factors for hypertension. Int J Mol Sci. 2018 Jun 11;19(6):1724.

22. Tangvoraphonkchai K, Davenport A. Magnesium and cardiovascular disease. Adv Chronic Kidney Dis. 2018 May;25(3):251–60.

23. Yang W, Omaye ST. Air pollutants, oxidative stress and human health. Mutat Res. 2009 Mar 31;674(1–2):45–54.

24. Calder PC. Nutrition, immunity and COVID-19. BMJ Nutr Prev Health. 2020 May 20;3(1):74–92.

25. Carr AC, Maggini S. Vitamin C and immune function. Nutrients. 2017 Nov 3;9(11):1211.

26. Pauling L. Vitamin C, the common cold and the flu. San Francisco: W.H. Freeman; 1976.

27. *Ibid.*

28. Malmgaard L. Induction and regulation of IFNs during viral infections. J Interferon Cytokine Res. 2004 Aug;24(8):439–54.

29. Kim Y, Kim H, Bae S, et al. Vitamin C is an essential factor on the anti-viral immune responses through the production of interferon-alpha/beta at the initial stage of influenza A virus (H3N2) infection. Immune Netw. 2013 Apr;13(2):70–74.

30. Marik PE, Hooper MH. Doctor—your septic patients have scurvy! Crit Care. 2018 Jan 29;22(1):23–24.

31. Hemmati AA, Nazari Z, Ranjbari N, et al. Comparison of the preventive effect of vitamin C and E on hexavalent chromium induced pulmonary fibrosis in rat. Inflammopharmacology. 2008 Aug;16(4): 195–97.

32. Holford P, Carr AC, Jovic TH, et al. Vitamin C—an adjunctive therapy for respiratory infection, sepsis and COVID-19. Nutrients. 2020 Dec 7;12(12): 3760.

33. Liu F, Zhu Y, Zhang J, et al. Intravenous high-dose vitamin C for the treatment of severe COVID-19: study protocol for a multicentre randomised controlled trial. BMJ Open. 2020 Jul 8;10(7):e039519.

34. Marik PE, Hooper MH. Doctor—your septic patients have scurvy! Crit Care. 2018 Jan 29;22(1):23–24.

35. Fiorino S, Gallo C, Zippi M, et al. Cytokine storm in aged people with CoV-2: possible role of vitamins as therapy or preventive strategy. Aging Clin Exp Res. 2020 Oct;32(10):2115–31.

36. Lytle CD, Sagripanti JL. Predicted inactivation of viruses of relevance to biodefense by solar radiation. J Virol. 2005 Nov;79(22):14244–52.

37. Beck MA, Handy J, Levander OA. Host nutritional status: the neglected virulence factor. Trends Microbiol. 2004 Sep;12(9):417–23.

38. *Ibid.*

39. *Ibid.*

40. Bakadia BM, Boni BOO, Ahmed AAQ, et al. The impact of oxidative stress damage induced by the environmental stressors on COVID-19. Life Sci. 2021 Jan 1;264:118653.

41. Palacios C, Gonzalez L. Is vitamin D deficiency a major global public health problem? J Steroid Biochem Mol Biol. 2014 Oct;144 Pt A:138–45.

42. Bruins MJ, Van Dael P, Eggersdorfer M. The role of nutrients in reducing the risk for noncommunicable diseases during aging. Nutrients. 2019 Jan 4; 11(1):85.

43. Jayanama K, Theou O, Blodgett JM, et al. Frailty, nutrition-related parameters, and mortality across the adult age spectrum. BMC Med. 2018 Oct 26;16(1):188.

44. Ellulu MS, Rahmat A, Patimah I, et al. Effect of vitamin C on inflammation and metabolic markers in hypertensive and/or diabetic obese adults: a randomized controlled trial. Drug Des Devel Ther. 2015 Jul 1;9:3405–12.

45. Afkhami-Ardekani M, Shojaoddiny-Ardekani A. Effect of vitamin C on blood glucose, serum lipids & serum insulin in type 2 diabetes patients. Indian J Med Res. 2007 Nov;126(5):471–74.

46. Zhou C, Na L, Shan R, et al. Dietary vitamin C intake reduces the risk of type 2 diabetes in Chinese adults: HOMA-IR and T-AOC as potential mediators. PLoS One. 2016 Sep 29;11(9):e0163571.

47. Fletcher RH, Fairfield KM. Vitamins for chronic disease prevention in adults: clinical applications. JAMA. 2002 Jun 19;287(23):3127–29.

48. Bicknell F, Prescott F. The vitamins in medicine. London: Heinemann; 1942. p. 3.

49. Fiorino S, Gallo C, Zippi M, et al. Cytokine storm in aged people with CoV-2: possible role of vitamins as therapy or preventive strategy. Aging Clin Exp Res. 2020 Oct;32(10):2115–31.

50. Calder PC. Nutrition, immunity and COVID-19. BMJ Nutr Prev Health. 2020 May 20;3(1):74–92.

51. Zed PJ, Abu-Laban RB, Balen RM, et al. Incidence, severity and preventability of medication-related visits to the emergency department: a prospective study. CMAJ. 2008 Jun 3;178(12):1563–69.

52. Cathcart RF. Vitamin C, titrating to bowel tolerance, anascorbemia, and acute induced scurvy. Med Hypotheses. 1981 Nov;7(11):1359–76.

53. Calder PC, Carr AC, Gombart AF, et al. Optimal nutritional status for a well-functioning immune system is an important factor to protect against viral infections. Nutrients. 2020 Apr 23;12(4):1181.

54. NIH Office of Dietary Supplements. Vitamin K: fact sheet for health professionals [Internet]. US Department of Health and Human Services; 2016. Available from: https://ods.od.nih.gov/factsheets/VitaminK-HealthProfessional.

55. Micronutrient Information Center. Vitamin B_{12} [Internet]. Corvallis (OR): Linus Pauling Institute, Oregon State University; 2015. Available from: http://lpi.oregonstate.edu/mic/vitamins/vitamin-B12.

56. Fulgoni VL 3rd, Keast DR, Bailey RI, et al. Foods, fortificants, and supplements: Where do Americans get their nutrients? J Nutr. 2011 Oct; 141(10):1847–54.

57. Kennedy DO. B vitamins and the brain: mechanisms, dose and efficacy—a review. Nutrients. 2016 Jan 27;8(2):68.

58. Biesalski HK, Tinz J. Multivitamin/mineral supplements: rationale and safety. Nutrition. 2017 Apr;36:60–66.

59. Robitaille L, Mamer OA, Miller WH Jr, et al. Oxalic acid excretion after intravenous ascorbic acid administration. Metabolism. 2009 Feb;58(2):263–69.

60. Holick MF, Chen TC. Vitamin D deficiency: a worldwide problem with health consequences. Am J Clin Nutr. 2008 Apr;87(4):1080S–6S.

61. Ahmed F. A network-based analysis reveals the mechanism underlying vitamin D in suppressing cytokine storm and virus in SARS-CoV-2 infection. Front Immunol. 2020 Dec 9;11:590459.

62. Cannell JJ, Hollis BW, Zasloff M, et al. Diagnosis and treatment of vitamin D deficiency. Expert Opin Pharmacother. 2008 Jan;9(1):107–18.

63. Žmitek K, Hribar M, Hristov H, et al. Efficiency of vitamin D supplementation in healthy adults is associated with body mass index and baseline serum 25-hydroxyvitamin D level. Nutrients. 2020 Apr 29;12(5):1268.

64. Lewis ED, Meydani SN, Wu D. Regulatory role of vitamin E in the immune system and inflammation. IUBMB Life. 2019 Apr;71(4):487–94.

65. Niki E, Noguchi N, Tsuchihashi H, et al. Interaction among vitamin C, vitamin E, and beta-carotene. Am J Clin Nutr. 1995 Dec;62 (6 Suppl): 1322S–26S.

66. Pickering G, Mazur A, Trousselard M, et al. Magnesium status and stress: the vicious circle concept revisited. Nutrients. 2020 Nov 28;12(12):3672.

67. Tang CF, Ding H, Jiao RQ, et al. Possibility of magnesium supplementation for supportive treatment in patients with COVID-19. Eur J Pharmacol. 2020 Nov 5;886:173546.

68. Gröber U, Schmidt J, Kisters K. Magnesium in prevention and therapy. Nutrients. 2015 Sep 23;7(9):8199–226.

69. Mori S, Tomita T, Fujimura K, et al. A randomized double-blind placebo-controlled trial on the effect of magnesium oxide in patients with chronic constipation. J Neurogastroenterol Motil. 2019 Oct 30;25(4):563–75.

70. Husson MO, Ley D, Portal C, et al. Modulation of host defence against bacterial and viral infections by omega-3 polyunsaturated fatty acids. J Infect. 2016 Dec;73(6):523–35.

71. Simopoulos AP. The importance of the ratio of omega-6/omega-3 essential fatty acids. Biomed Pharmacother. 2002 Oct;56(8):365–79.

72. Langlois PL, D'Aragon F, Hardy G, et al. Omega-3 polyunsaturated fatty acids in critically ill patients with acute respiratory distress syndrome: a systematic review and meta-analysis. Nutrition. 2019 May;61:84–92.

73. Timoneda J, Rodríguez-Fernández L, Zaragozá R, et al. Vitamin A deficiency and the lung. Nutrients. 2018 Aug 21;10(9):1132.

74. Semba RD, Muhilal, Scott AL, et al. Depressed immune response to tetanus in children with vitamin A deficiency. J Nutr. 1992 Jan;122(1):101–7.

75. Institute of Medicine (US) Panel on Micronutrients. Vitamin K [Internet]. Dietary reference intakes for vitamin a, vitamin k, arsenic, boron, chromium, copper, iodine, iron, manganese, molybdenum, nickel, silicon, vanadium, and zinc. US National Library of Medicine; 1970. Available from: https://www.ncbi.nlm.nih.gov/books/NBK222299/.

76. Janssen R, Visser MPJ, Dofferhoff ASM, et al. Vitamin K metabolism as the potential missing link between lung damage and thromboembolism in Coronavirus disease 2019. Br J Nutr. 2020 Oct 7:1–8.

Epilogue: Looking Back; Thinking Forward

1. Raisi-Estabragh Z, McCracken C, Bethell MS, et al. Greater risk of severe COVID-19 in Black, Asian and Minority Ethnic populations is not explained by cardiometabolic, socioeconomic or behavioural factors, or by 25(OH)-vitamin D status: study of 1326 cases from the UK Biobank. J Public Health (Oxf). 2020 Aug 18;42(3):451–60.

2. COVID-19—What we know so far about . . . social determinants of health [Internet]. Public Health Ontario; 2020 May 24. Available from: https://www.publichealthontario.ca/-/media/documents/ncov/covid-wwksf/2020/05/what-we-know-social-determinants-health.pdf.

3. Whiting SJ, Langlois KA, Vatanparast H, et al. The vitamin D status of Canadians relative to the 2011 Dietary Reference Intakes: an examination in children and adults with and without supplement use. Am J Clin Nutr. 2011 Jul;94(1):128–35.

4. D'Amore R. Vitamin D and COVID-19: experts say any possible link is "premature" [Internet]. Global News; 2020 Jul 30. Available from: https://globalnews.ca/news/7229458/coronavirus-vitamin-d-studies.

5. Di Rosa M, Malaguarnera M, Nicoletti F. Vitamin D3: a helpful immuno-modulator. Immunology 2011;134(2):123–39.

6. Treatments [Internet]. BC Centre for Disease Control; updated 2021 Jan 29. Available from: http://www.bccdc.ca/health-professionals/clinical-resources/covid-19-care/clinical-care/treatments.

7. Roberts S. The Swiss cheese model of pandemic defense [Internet]. New York Times; 2020 Dec 5. Available from: https://www.nytimes.com/2020/12/05/health/coronavirus-swiss-cheese-infection-mackay.html.

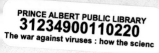